THE THREAT OF AND PLANNING FOR PANDEMIC FLU

HEARING

BEFORE THE

SUBCOMMITTEE ON HEALTH

OF THE

COMMITTEE ON ENERGY AND COMMERCE

HOUSE OF REPRESENTATIVES

ONE HUNDRED NINTH CONGRESS

FIRST SESSION

MAY 26, 2005

Serial No. 109–21

Printed for the use of the Committee on Energy and Commerce

Available via the World Wide Web: http://www.access.gpo.gov/congress/house

U.S. GOVERNMENT PRINTING OFFICE

21–642PDF

WASHINGTON : 2005

COMMITTEE ON ENERGY AND COMMERCE

JOE BARTON, Texas, *Chairman*

RALPH M. HALL, Texas
MICHAEL BILIRAKIS, Florida
  Vice Chairman
FRED UPTON, Michigan
CLIFF STEARNS, Florida
PAUL E. GILLMOR, Ohio
NATHAN DEAL, Georgia
ED WHITFIELD, Kentucky
CHARLIE NORWOOD, Georgia
BARBARA CUBIN, Wyoming
JOHN SHIMKUS, Illinois
HEATHER WILSON, New Mexico
JOHN B. SHADEGG, Arizona
CHARLES W. "CHIP" PICKERING,
  Mississippi, *Vice Chairman*
VITO FOSSELLA, New York
ROY BLUNT, Missouri
STEVE BUYER, Indiana
GEORGE RADANOVICH, California
CHARLES F. BASS, New Hampshire
JOSEPH R. PITTS, Pennsylvania
MARY BONO, California
GREG WALDEN, Oregon
LEE TERRY, Nebraska
MIKE FERGUSON, New Jersey
MIKE ROGERS, Michigan
C.L. "BUTCH" OTTER, Idaho
SUE MYRICK, North Carolina
JOHN SULLIVAN, Oklahoma
TIM MURPHY, Pennsylvania
MICHAEL C. BURGESS, Texas
MARSHA BLACKBURN, Tennessee

JOHN D. DINGELL, Michigan
  Ranking Member
HENRY A. WAXMAN, California
EDWARD J. MARKEY, Massachusetts
RICK BOUCHER, Virginia
EDOLPHUS TOWNS, New York
FRANK PALLONE, Jr., New Jersey
SHERROD BROWN, Ohio
BART GORDON, Tennessee
BOBBY L. RUSH, Illinois
ANNA G. ESHOO, California
BART STUPAK, Michigan
ELIOT L. ENGEL, New York
ALBERT R. WYNN, Maryland
GENE GREEN, Texas
TED STRICKLAND, Ohio
DIANA DeGETTE, Colorado
LOIS CAPPS, California
MIKE DOYLE, Pennsylvania
TOM ALLEN, Maine
JIM DAVIS, Florida
JAN SCHAKOWSKY, Illinois
HILDA L. SOLIS, California
CHARLES A. GONZALEZ, Texas
JAY INSLEE, Washington
TAMMY BALDWIN, Wisconsin
MIKE ROSS, Arkansas

BUD ALBRIGHT, *Staff Director*
DAVID CAVICKE, *Deputy Staff Director and General Counsel*
REID P.F. STUNTZ, *Minority Staff Director and Chief Counsel*

SUBCOMMITTEE ON HEALTH

NATHAN DEAL, Georgia, *Chairman*

RALPH M. HALL, Texas
MICHAEL BILIRAKIS, Florida
FRED UPTON, Michigan
PAUL E. GILLMOR, Ohio
CHARLIE NORWOOD, Georgia
BARBARA CUBIN, Wyoming
JOHN SHIMKUS, Illinois
JOHN B. SHADEGG, Arizona
CHARLES W. "CHIP" PICKERING,
  Mississippi
STEVE BUYER, Indiana
JOSEPH R. PITTS, Pennsylvania
MARY BONO, California
MIKE FERGUSON, New Jersey
MIKE ROGERS, Michigan
SUE MYRICK, North Carolina
MICHAEL C. BURGESS, Texas
JOE BARTON, Texas,
  (Ex Officio)

SHERROD BROWN, Ohio
  Ranking Member
HENRY A. WAXMAN, California
EDOLPHUS TOWNS, New York
FRANK PALLONE, Jr., New Jersey
BART GORDON, Tennessee
BOBBY L. RUSH, Illinois
ANNA G. ESHOO, California
GENE GREEN, Texas
TED STRICKLAND, Ohio
DIANA DeGETTE, Colorado
LOIS CAPPS, California
TOM ALLEN, Maine
JIM DAVIS, Florida
TAMMY BALDWIN, Wisconsin
JOHN D. DINGELL, Michigan,
  (Ex Officio)

CONTENTS

Page

(III)

THE THREAT OF AND PLANNING FOR PANDEMIC FLU

THURSDAY, MAY 26, 2005

House of Representatives,
Committee on Energy and Commerce,
Subcommittee on Health,
Washington, DC.

The subcommittee met, pursuant to notice, at 10:05 a.m., in room 2123 of the Rayburn House Office Building, Hon. Nathan Deal (chairman) presiding.

Members present: Representatives Deal, Hall, Shadegg, Pitts, Bono, Ferguson, Burgess, Barton (ex officio), Brown, Waxman, Eshoo, Green, DeGette, Allen, and Baldwin.

Staff present: Chuck Clapton, chief health counsel; Ryan Long, professional staff; Nandan Kenkermath, majority counsel; Eugenia Edwards, legislative clerk; Brandon Clark, health policy coordinator; John Ford, minority counsel; and Jessica McNiece, research assistant.

Mr. DEAL. Call to order. Please close the doors in the back and we will get started. The Chair recognizes himself for an opening statement.

I certainly want to welcome everyone to this hearing today and our distinguished panel members. We have two panels that you are going to hear from, and they will give various perspectives on this issue of pandemic flu. And certainly it is an issue that everybody, I suppose, has their own point of view on. And we will hear several points of view, I am sure, during the course of this hearing today.

Our first panel of witnesses contain some faces and names that are familiar to many of the members of this subcommittee. First of all, Dr. Julie Gerberding, who is now a fellow North Georgian, and I was going to brag about that until I heard from Mr. Brown as to where you graduated from medical school, so he is going to claim some credit for you as well. But being from the CDC in Atlanta and the director of that facility, I am certainly pleased to have you here today. Dr. Bruce Gellin, who is the director of the National Vaccine Program Office within the Department of Health and Human Services, pleased to have you, Dr. Gellin. And Dr. Anthony Fauci, who is the director of the National Institute of Allergy and Infectious Diseases within NIH. We are certainly pleased to have all three of you here today.

I am going to go ahead and introduce at this point the second panel, and I have to extend an apology probably that I won't be here for all of the second panel's testimony, but I might if I don't have too many long-winded opening statements here. I do have an engagement that is going to take me out for a while, but our vice-chairman will be presiding at that time.

Dr. Marcia Crosse, who is the director of Health Care Issues for the U.S. Government Accountability Office; Dr. Ralph Tripp, who is the director for the Center for Disease Intervention at the University of Georgia College of Veterinary Medicine and the Georgia Research Alliance Chair of the Animal Health Vaccine Development, and the second Georgian who is in the panel group today; Dr. Andrew Pavia, who is chair of the Taskforce on Pandemic Influenza at the Infectious Diseases Society of America; and professor and chief of the Division of Pediatric Infectious Diseases at University of Utah Health Services Center and Primary Children's Hospital; Dr. Dominick Iacuzio, close I am sure, medical director of the Hoffmann-La Roche, Incorporated; Mr. Phillip Hosbach, who is vice president of the Immunization Policy and Government Relations for sanofi pasteur, which is the world's largest influenza vaccine manufacturers.

So as you can see from the titles and the positions of the members of these two panels, we certainly represent, I think, a cross-section of the experts on this issue that we are facing today.

All of us, I think, can attest to the fact that the fear of a global influenza epidemic or a flu pandemic is certainly one of the greater health challenges and threats that our country faces and our world faces. All of us have different perspectives on this. I have heard people, as we have talked about having a hearing like this, saying that they remembered the Asian Flu, they remembered the flu epidemics when they were in college, and all of these things.

I have a resource that goes far beyond that, so I decided to ask my 98-year-old mother and my soon-to-be 92-year-old father-in-law what they remember about flu epidemics. And remarkably, my mother, who was a young teenager in the 1918 flu epidemic, recalls that she lost two aunts during that time. And those of you who know the history of all this, this was a serious flu that affected our country and affected the world.

My father-in-law went back even further than that. He remembered a flu epidemic of the late 1800's and recalled that there is a cemetery in our area where it is practically filled with the victims of a flu from the late 1800's. So the idea that this is something that is new is certainly not appropriate because it is a threat that has hit our country and the world in the past and is certainly a threat that we want to be sure that we are as prepared as we possibly can be.

You might ask why the linkage with the veterinary testimony. Part of it is the fact that my hometown calls itself the poultry capital of the world, and we have for many, many years, of course, been concerned with Avian Flu and the effects on the poultry industry here and across the world. But there is a direct linkage, as you will hear, in the threat and trying to eliminate the threat within the poultry and fowl of the world so that there is no transmission. So there is a linkage and we certainly want to hear about that today.

With that, again, I welcome all of you and we look forward to your testimony. And I will recognize my good friend, Mr. Brown.

[The prepared statement of Hon. Nathan Deal follows:]

PREPARED STATEMENT OF HON. NATHAN DEAL, CHAIRMAN, SUBCOMMITTEE ON HEALTH

The Committee will come to order, and the Chair recognizes himself for an opening statement.

I am proud to say that we have two expert panels of witnesses appearing before us today that I believe will fairly represent the different perspectives on this complex issue. We look forward to hearing your testimony, and we are grateful for your cooperation and attendance at today's hearing.

Our first panel of witnesses contains a few familiar faces to this Committee:

- Dr. Julie Gerberding, fellow North Georgia resident and Director of the Centers for Disease Control and Prevention.
- Dr. Bruce Gellin, Director of the National Vaccine Program Office within the Department of Health and Human Services
- Dr. Anthony Fauci, Director of the National Institute of Allergy and Infectious Diseases within National Institutes of Health

Our second panel comes to us largely from outside of the federal government and contains five experts witnesses:

- Dr. Marcia Crosse, Director of Health Care Issues for the U.S. Government Accountability Office
- Dr. Ralph Tripp, Director of the Center for Disease Intervention at the University of Georgia College of Veterinary Medicine and Georgia Research Alliance Chair of Animal Health Vaccine Development and our second witness hailing from North Georgia.
- Dr. Andrew Pavia, Chair of the Task Force on Pandemic Influenza at the Infectious Diseases Society of America and professor and chief of the Division of Pediatric Infectious Diseases at the University of Utah Health Sciences Center and Primary Children's Hospital
- Dr. Dominick Iacuzio, Medical Director for Hoffmann-La Roche, Inc.
- Mr. Phillip Hosbach, Vice President of Immunization Policy and Government Relations for Sanofi Pasteur, which is the world's largest influenza vaccine manufacturer

As all of our witnesses today will attest, the threat of a global influenza epidemic, or "flu pandemic," is one of the greatest public health threats we face today. From speaking to the experts in this field, I truly believe that it is not a matter of "if" a flu pandemic hits but "when," and I believe that is our responsibility as Members of Congress to ensure that the public is as protected from this threat as possible. This, of course, is no simple matter and there is no silver-bullet solution to this problem.

Protecting the public from the threat of a global flu pandemic takes awareness of the potential threat as well as dedication and cooperation from all of the involved organizations in both the public and private sectors. Unfortunately, I believe we have ignored the lessons of history and science and that we remain under prepared for the emergence of a global flu pandemic that could potentially kill millions of people over a short period of time and have irreparable harm to our economy.

As most of you know, I live in Gainesville, Georgia, which is considered to be the "Poultry Capital of the World," and each year my Congressional district produces over $915 million in farmgate value from the poultry industry. If we were struck by a virulent strain of the avian influenza virus, this entire industry would be completely wiped out in matter of weeks.

Clearly, we have too much at stake to continue to largely ignore this serious threat facing our society, and that is why I am excited about the opportunity we have before us today to further explore the potential threat of a pandemic flu and how we can better prepare to ourselves to face this problem.

I am a great believer in the potential of science and human determination and I firmly believe that if we dedicate ourselves and our resources to solving this problem that we can overcome this significant threat looming on our horizon.

Again, I welcome our witnesses and thank them for their participation. I now recognize my friend from Ohio, Mr. Brown, for five minutes for his opening statement.

Mr. BROWN. Thank you, Mr. Chairman. Thank you to all three witnesses, frankly, three of the most important people in our government and our country. We welcome you to share your wisdom with us and to thank you for your public service and the terrific work you do for our healthcare system and especially for our public health infrastructure.

In March, during a hearing on the National Institutes of Health, the director showed the committee a slide charting the increase and life expectancy in the United States over the last century. That slide illustrated a number of things, including the progress our country made in developing our public health infrastructure and expanding healthcare coverage and access, especially for seniors, and in fostering breakthroughs in biomedical research.

Perhaps the most notable thing on the chart—other than the 30-year growth in life expectancy brought on mostly by public health, secondarily by major high-tech medical breakthroughs—but perhaps the most notable thing on the chart was the downward spike in the year 1918. The last major pandemic flu infected 28 percent of Americans, caused the deaths of nearly 700,000 people, as we know; worldwide killed in excess of 25 million people; some estimate as high as 50 million, more than the first World War that ended that same year. Life expectancy in our country dropped 12 years in 12 months. The example of the early 20th century remains relevant today as a warning to public health experts, to government officials, including Members of this Congress who have absolutely inadequately funded public health.

1918 shows how the spread of a flu strain that evades available treatment lurks as one of the most serious risks to our Nation's health. Our Nation and the international community of which we remain vulnerable to flu strains that evade available treatment and, as I said, can potentially wreak havoc on the Nation's public health, obviously there are important differences between 1918 and 2005. Many of those differences are reflected in the makeup of our two panels today because of the coordination and research led by CDC and NIH, our ability to identify, prevent, and fight potentially harmful infection is far superior to where we were early last century.

But along with this progress we face new challenges—a world with seamless and constant global travel makes an outbreak in the remotest corner of the world a threat to every corner. When infection travels to Hong Kong to Hartford in a matter of hours, it becomes significantly harder, obviously, to contain.

Manmade treatments save millions but inadequate and misapplied therapies have fostered new drug-resistant strains of infection, especially a disease like tuberculosis. We have seen a number of potential vaccine suppliers dwindle into the single digits, and without adequate funding at the Federal, State, and local level in large part because of decisions on tax cuts and spending priorities made in this Congress, our public health infrastructure is woefully unprepared to fight a major outbreak and to deal with daily problems in public health, in the deaths and the illnesses of people who most of us on this panel, frankly, don't know—people in the inner city, people afflicted by rural poverty.

These challenges resonated loudly last fall when it was announced the U.S. would short nearly half of our expected flu vaccine. I admire the word done by HHS and CDC to inform the public and develop guidelines in the face of that shortage, but we must apply the lessons learned last year and do it now. We don't know whether we will face a pandemic, but we do know that countless lives could be loss of a pandemic takes hold.

Epidemiologists and other public health experts are currently tracking several potential flu pandemics, the Avian Influenza, or Bird Flu, appears to pose the most lethal threat. As of March, Avian Flu had killed 74 people in Asian and tens of millions of birds. The global threat is a potential for the virus to mutate and spread from human to human. The World Health Organization has said that because of that possibility the world is "closer to an influenza pandemic than in any time since 1968." WHO further points out similarities that suggest Avian Flu could follow the same patterns as the strain that caused the 1918 pandemic. The threat posed by Avian Flu is great, but with the right investment and collaboration from industry, academia, and government, a pandemic can be averted. This committee should consider how best to ensure the development, stockpile, and distribution of vaccine and antiviral treatments. It must examine the avenues government can take to bring competition and diversity back into the vaccine market, ideally before a pandemic strain could hit our shores. We should continue to work with partners like WHO to fight infection where it exists and prevent worldwide transmission. We should examine our Nation's investment in basic research and better understand how that commitment translates into more effective remedies for potential pandemic. We should go beyond a discussion of pandemic flu and talk about how and how much and how we should fund our public health infrastructure, not just for major outbreaks that will affect everyone, but the kind of day-to-day public health that, frankly, the public health problems that our Congress and our government, frankly, have so far been unwilling to address. Thank you, Mr. Chairman.

Mr. DEAL. We are pleased to have the chairman of our full committee, Mr. Barton from Texas, and I recognize him at this time for an opening statement.

Chairman BARTON. Thank you, Mr. Chairman. I want to commend you for holding this hearing. I want to commend both of our panels of witnesses, the first panel and the second panel, for being here on this important subject.

There are experts that say another killer flu epidemic is inevitable. We don't know when or where it will begin or exactly how many million that it will kill; we only know that a pandemic flu has happened before, and we think that it almost surely will happen again. Historically, influenza pandemics have been deadly. With a world population of six-and-a-half billion, even a relatively mild pandemic could kill millions of people. In the United States the risk varies from tens of thousands to hundreds of thousands. Put it like this: a bad flu outbreak could kill more Americans than either or both of the last two World Wars. It is probably fair to expect that some of us in this room today would be sick and possibly a handful of the people in this room would even die.

Right now we are monitoring some serious developments in Asia concerning the recent Avian Flu strain. Both the World Health Organization and the Department of Health and Human Services has expressed serious concerns over these strains developing into a global pandemic. Organizations around the world and Health and Human Services in our country have taken significant steps to mitigate the potential effects of influenza pandemic.

That is the purpose of the hearing today is to do oversight on those steps. I want to applaud the efforts in this country in both the private sector and the public sector. I also want to applaud the Secretary of Health and Human Services for his emphasis on planning and preparedness for a pandemic flu and his cooperation with international organizations.

In many other ways we do remain vulnerable. The global vaccine industry is fragile. The capacity to gear up and produce the necessary vaccines in the event of a pandemic is limited. Liability concerns may hinder production and distribution of any new vaccine. With ordinary flu vaccine production already so low, the amounts that we can produce in the face of a global pandemic are probably insufficient. Moreover, the timeframes for development, production, and approvals leave millions and millions of people vulnerable. Antivirals may also be a countermeasure. We can place such countermeasures in the national strategic stockpile, and I am glad that we have done so with over two millions courses of treatment so far.

But one question that we need to try to get an answer for today is whether this is sufficient in the face of the apparent threat. The amount in relation to population would appear to be much less than what other countries are doing. I would also note that many similar planning and preparedness activities will be relevant in the face of bioterrorism and other emerging threats. We need to work aggressively and cooperatively on all of these issues.

Again, Mr. Chairman, thank you for the hearing. I look forward to hearing from our witnesses today. And with that I yield back.

[The prepared statement of Hon. Joe Barton follows:]

PREPARED STATEMENT OF HON. JOE BARTON, CHAIRMAN, COMMITTEE ON ENERGY AND COMMERCE

Thank you, Mr. Chairman. I commend you for holding this hearing on this important public health issue.

Experts say another killer flu is inevitable. We don't know when or where it will begin, or exactly how many millions it may kill. We only know that a pandemic flu has happened before and it must surely come again. Historically, influenza pandemics have been deadly. With a world population of 6.5 billion, even a relatively mild pandemic could kill many millions of people. In the United States the risk varies from tens of thousands to hundreds of thousands. Think of it like this—a bad flu outbreak could kill more Americans than either or both of the last century's world wars. It is probably fair to expect that some of us in this room today would be sick, and a handful of us would die.

Right now we are monitoring some serious developments in Asia concerning a recent avian flu strain. Both the World Health Organization and the Department of Health and Human Services has expressed serious concern over these strains developing into a global pandemic.

Organizations around the world and HHS have taken significant steps to mitigate the potential effects of influenza pandemic. I applaud the efforts that both the private sector and public sector are making to address the potential need for different means of vaccine production. I also applaud the Secretary of HHS for the emphasis on planning and preparedness for pandemic flu and cooperation with international organizations.

In many other ways, however, we remain very vulnerable. The global vaccine industry is fragile and sparse. The capacity to gear up and produce necessary vaccines in the event of a pandemic is limited. Liability concerns may hinder production and distribution of any new vaccine. With ordinary flu vaccine production so low, the amounts we can produce in the face of a global pandemic are insufficient. Moreover, the time frames for development, production, and approvals leave millions vulnerable.

Antivirals may also be a useful countermeasure. We can place such countermeasures in the National Strategic Stockpile. I am glad we have done so for over

2 million courses of treatment, but I want to ask whether this is sufficient in the face of the threat. The amount in relation to the population appears to be much less than what other countries are doing.

I note that many similar planning and preparedness activities will be relevant in the face of bioterrorism and other emerging threats. We will need to aggressively work on these issues. I look forward to hearing from today's witnesses on this timely and important topic.

Mr. DEAL. Thank you, Mr. Chairman. I am pleased to recognize the gentlelady from California, Ms. Eshoo, for an opening statement.

Ms. ESHOO. Thank you, Mr. Chairman, and good morning to you and welcome to our very distinguished panel. It is always a pleasure when you come to the committee to testify and I salute you for your work on behalf of the American people. I think you always distinguish yourselves.

The World Health Organization has warned that a pandemic flu could occur at any time, which could cause deaths—as has been stated by some of my colleagues already—in a range of two to seven million people. Those are staggering numbers. I can't help but think of—I don't know whether it was in the 1970's or 1980's—we saw something very common on people's desks, and it said "plan"—and then "ahead" kind of just fell off the edge. So I think that today we are trying to plan ahead and be wise, be prudent, and understand the factors that really didn't come into play with the flu epidemic that we had in our own country, the shortcomings that occurred, the lurch that people found themselves in. And the best question that people asked from senior centers and medical centers across the country was why were we not prepared for this? Why hasn't this worked?

The Avian Flu, known as the Bird Flu, is the latest strain of concern. Should it adapt fully to humans and be capable of easy person-to-person transmission, it would probably spread worldwide in 3 to 6 months.

Right now only about a dozen companies in the world make flu vaccines. Many of these manufacturers are based overseas. This is a serious problem for the United States if and when a pandemic hits. In a pandemic, overseas manufacturers may be reluctant to provide the United States with their stockpile, and if they do agree to provide us with the vaccines, the FDA will need the ability to rapidly evaluate the vaccine or agree to let them in automatically once they are approved.

We also know that it is financially risky for manufacturers to invest in research and development because the pandemic strain that emerges may be substantially different from any vaccine in development. There could likely be an investment without any return.

So the Congress has to take steps to ensure that there is a robust infrastructure for developing and providing vaccines and treatments. We have to address the barriers that manufacturers face. Today, I hope HHS will explain why their draft pandemic flu plan is still not final, and I hope that the CDC can explain why there has been a delay in stockpiling antivirals, which, if taken within 2 days of getting sick, can reduce the symptoms of the flu and shorten the time that one is sick by 1 or 2 days. Antivirals can make one less contagious to others.

So I look forward to the testimony from our expert panels on this issue, and I hope that this committee will act quickly and appropriately to prepare for pandemic flu. The American people are counting on us to do that. Thank you, Mr. Chairman, for holding this important hearing.

Mr. DEAL. Thank you. I recognize the vice-chairman of the subcommittee, Mr. Ferguson, for an opening statement.

Mr. FERGUSON. Thank you, Mr. Chairman. Thank you for holding this hearing and I thank our two panels of distinguished guests today. I am looking forward to hearing their testimony.

Mr. Chairman, we are staring down the barrel of a loaded gun, and that gun is ready to fire. Expert after expert, including the esteemed witnesses that we will hear from today, have said that we must not ask if but when. When will we face the strain of influenza virus that will cause a pandemic? And when that happens, will we be ready?

We have heard these figures before but they are important to repeat. In 1918 an influenza pandemic claimed the lives of almost 600,000 Americans and more than 20 million people worldwide. A little known fact to most people is that in a regular flu season today kills about 36,000 Americans. Today, public health experts at HHS and CDC estimate that an influenza pandemic could cause 90,000 to 300,000 or more deaths in the U.S. and tens of millions of people worldwide. Pandemic influenza is nature's weapon of mass destruction. Even the Homeland Security Department has weighed in on a flu pandemic's effects, pegging the cost of a pandemic influenza outbreak in just four cities in the United States at $70 billion to $160 billion.

Dr. Michael Osterholm, head of University of Minnesota's Center for Infectious Disease Research and Police stated in the "Wall Street Journal" just this week that a pandemic flu could trigger an economic crisis. Dr. Osterholm noted that the 2003 outbreak of SARS paralyzed cities and cost billions of dollars even though its toll, 8,000 sick and 800 dead, was relatively light. Pandemic flu could change the world overnight, Dr. Osterholm stated, reducing or even ending foreign travel and trade.

This problem demands our full attention and the full commitment of our resources to counter a looming catastrophe. Last November this Health Subcommittee held hearings as last year's flu season was underway. Just a few weeks ago the Oversight and Investigations Subcommittee held a perspective hearing on the upcoming flu season and what we are doing to ramp up vaccine production. But this hearing will be looking at the threat of pandemic flu and our vital surveillance efforts of Avian Flu strains in Asia, what is being done to ramp up vaccine capacity once a pandemic strain is identified, and what the response plan is while a pandemic is occurring, specifically preparedness through stockpiling antivirals.

In each of the hearings we have had on the flu I have stressed the importance of stockpiling antivirals to treat those who are infected with the flu. Antivirals are a potent way to combat a flu outbreak and are unique compared to vaccines because they can be stockpiled for between 5 to 7 years, or perhaps more.

I look forward to hearing from our distinguished panels today. I look forward to hearing their insight on how we can be best prepared when the feared pandemic does in fact strike. Thank you, Mr. Chairman. I yield back.

Mr. DEAL. Thank you. Pleased to recognize gentlelady from Colorado, Ms. DeGette, for an opening statement.

Ms. DeGETTE. Thank you, Mr. Chairman. Simply to say how much I appreciate you having this important hearing. I will submit my opening statement for the record and reserve my time for questions.

Mr. DEAL. I thank the gentlelady. Chair recognizes Dr. Burgess for an opening statement.

Mr. BURGESS. Thank you, Mr. Chairman, and I too want to thank you for calling this hearing and thank the full committee chairman and the ranking member for holding this hearing.

Looking at the historical significance of pandemic flu, it is almost overwhelming to think about the challenges of preventing a devastating outbreak of influenza and dealing with the aftermath. The numbers are significant. In the last century it is estimated that over 53 million people died from periodic outbreaks of pandemic flu strains. Considering the world's population is much more mobile today than at any time in our history, I think the public health officials are right in making the fight against communicable disease one of their highest priorities. If we factor in the adaptability of the influenza virus and the fact that an airplane makes a pretty good way to communicate an illness like the flu, it is understandable to see why we cannot consign the pandemic flu outbreaks of the last century to the will-not-recur file.

There are tools available to us to confront a possible outbreak, but the coordination, the surveillance, and the prevention of a containment strategy are going to affect us at the State, Federal, and, yes, at the global levels. The severity of the next pandemic cannot be predicted, but even a medium-level pandemic could cause between 100,000 and 200,000 deaths, almost three-quarters of a million hospitalizations, and millions and millions of people in doctors' offices, outpatient visits, and missing work. An estimated economic impact would be well over $150 billion for a medium outbreak.

Not too long ago we were concerned about another communicable disease, SARS virus. The SARS outbreak of 2003 exposed the capability of global surveillance and the containment infrastructure as to how an outbreak of an unknown disease can impact human interaction and commerce. And, Dr. Gerberding, I thank you for tolerating my many phone calls over that period. But even though the severity of the outbreak was largely isolated to East and South Asian countries, it did impact my district, which at the time was the home to the Dallas/Fort Worth Airport. At the local level at least, the SARS outbreak brought into sharp focus how fear can drive a containment response to an illness in the absence of a workable containment strategy.

The chairman brought up about the issue of liability and the ranking member brought up about how we can assure the development and availability of vaccines, and I too believe that somehow controlling liability in the manufacture and production of vaccines is going to be critical in our ability to provide this on a larger scale.

But I look forward to hearing our panel today, and I understand that our current capabilities of our public health institutions and the vaccine industry will help improve our response to any further pandemic outbreaks. Mr. Chairman, thank you again, and I will yield back my time.

Mr. DEAL. Thank you. Recognize the gentleman from Maine, Mr. Allen.

Mr. ALLEN. Thank you, Mr. Chairman. I appreciate your calling this hearing to examine the level of U.S. preparedness for a possible flu pandemic. I look forward to hearing from our expert witnesses on our current level of preparedness.

Unlike past flu pandemics, the relatively gradual emergence of the Avian Bird Flu has given us time to ensure that we have adequate resources to fight this deadly virus. At this point we don't know when or if the current strain of Avian Bird Flu will reach the U.S., but we do know that the epidemiology of the H5N1 virus is more virulent and has already passed directly from human to human. We know that this particular flu strain has infected at least 92 adults in Vietnam, Thailand, and Cambodia killing 52 people. We also know that there is currently no vaccine for Avian Flu and no known cure.

I am concerned about our country's ability to develop, approve, and secure adequate vaccine supplies. Today the U.S. has one domestic source of flu vaccine. America has been a world leader in developing life-saving medicines and spearheading countless global health efforts. April 12, 2005 marked the 50th anniversary of the first polio vaccine. Polio was eliminated in the U.S. because protecting the public's health was perceived as a simple necessity, and every effort was made to see that the vaccine would be freely distributed and polio would be eradicated. Without diligent efforts to maintain immunization programs here and strengthen them worldwide, we would not be able to keep such deadly diseases at bay.

The spread of the H5N1 virus poses a new challenge to the U.S. scientific community and vaccine manufacturers. Many experts have stated that we need a more reliable and flexible vaccine production system, as well as improved surveillance and public communication. Last year the license suspension of the Chiron Company's vaccine manufacturing plant in the U.K. served as a wake-up call. In addition to a shortage of supply, we were faced with trying to educate the public about appropriate distribution and who should be vaccinated first.

It is my understanding that countries such as Canada, Japan, Australia, and New Zealand are stockpiling antiviral treatments against pandemic flu for up to one-quarter of their nation's population. The U.S. stockpile is currently maintained for only 1 percent of our population, and I believe this strategy needs to be reexamined.

I hope the witnesses will help us understand what went wrong last year and what we can do to strengthen our domestic vaccine supply, speed research and development, and establish better distribution channels. Thank you again, Mr. Chairman, and I yield back.

Mr. DEAL. I thank the gentleman. Chair recognizes Mr. Shadegg for an opening statement.

Mr. SHADEGG. Thank you, Mr. Chairman, and thank you for holding this important hearing on this topic. As my colleagues have already noted, a pandemic flu could pose a very serious health threat to not only our country but to the world. But it should also be noted that it could also lead to an economic crisis. Just yesterday a "Wall Street Journal" article noted that "A pandemic flu could sicken more than a billion people and single-handedly stop travel and trade throughout the world, resulting in untold economic losses." We have spent considerable time and resources over the past few years preparing for an attack of bioterrorism. Now, the lessons learned from that experience should be used to address pandemic flu.

The first and foremost of these lessons is that our best defense is a strong offense. Preventing outbreaks through vaccine development will ensure that a flu eruption fails to reach pandemic status. I want to thank our witnesses for their work and for their efforts to ensure that vaccines prevent pandemic flu outbreaks, as well as for their testimony on what we can do to meet the goals that we have set.

We also must be prepared, however, for an outbreak that cannot be addressed through vaccination. In such an instance we must have adequate surveillance systems to ensure early recognition, sufficient communication tools, and networks to enable response, and antiviral providers able to respond.

Again, Mr. Chairman, I thank you for sponsoring this hearing and for your efforts in this regard. And I thank our witnesses for their testimony and their work in this area.

Mr. DEAL. Thank you. Recognize Ms. Baldwin for an opening statement.

Ms. BALDWIN. Thank you, Mr. Chairman. I too want to commend you for holding this hearing today. I was wondering last night as I began to read through the materials whether I would be kept up all night by the dire threats. And as many of my colleagues have noted, pandemic flu poses a serious threat to our Nation and the world. A recent article in the science publication "Nature" notes that a flu pandemic could cause 20 percent of the world's population to become sick, almost 30 million may need to be hospitalized, and a quarter of those infected would die. And perhaps the most shocking aspect of that article was that experts cited considered those numbers optimistic.

Many experts are now saying that a pandemic flu occurring in the United States is not a question of if but when. And in our day of globalization when it takes mere hours to cross continents, the old ways of containing an infectious disease are no longer applicable.

While I am glad that the Department of Health and Human Services has produced a draft of the Pandemic Influenza Preparedness and Response Plan, I remain concerned about the lack of progress on finalizing the report, and particularly, in light of our crisis last fall when the delivery of vaccine for seasonal flu was severely curtailed and only guidelines and voluntary opting out by more healthy individuals helped us address that crisis. It is imperative, I think, that we move quickly and decisively, and we have some catching up to do.

I also note that experts stress again and again that our planning efforts must be international in scope and look forward to hearing from witnesses today on that aspect of our planning efforts. There are several other aspects of our preparedness that I hope to hear you address through your testimony this morning. For example, I think we need to start educating Americans, not just healthcare providers, but American citizens need to know what to do in the case of an outbreak, what their treatment and prevent options are, which authorities to go to for information and what medications could be available to them should an outbreak occur.

I also hope to hear your thoughts on the importance of seamless communication, information sharing, and access to resources among our healthcare professionals. The chain will be only as strong as our weakest length and a public health nurse in a rural county in Wisconsin must have the same access to resources as a public health nurse in midtown Manhattan. Groups and regions ought not to be place in competition with each other.

If a pandemic flu should occur in the U.S., there will be a terrific strain on our ability to provide medications as well as treatments in our clinics and hospitals. If high numbers of people get sick, who will decide who gets care in a hospital when all the beds are full? Who gets placed in the ICU? Who gets the last dose of an antiviral medication?

I look forward to hearing the witnesses today tackle some of these very challenging questions. Thank you, Mr. Chairman. I yield back.

Mr. DEAL. Thank you. I too share the lady's concern. These are rather frightening statistics. And from this point forward nobody in the audience is allowed to cough, and if you do, the hypochondriacs in our midst are going to leave the room. So I am pleased to recognize Mr. Hall for an opening statement.

Mr. HALL. Mr. Chairman, thank you. And you would never get Howard Hughes to shake hands with any of us here today, would you? I thank you and I join the accolades of the other members here to the Chair for holding this hearing and for other hearings that he is very capable of holding and has held for this committee and for this Congress.

You know, listening to the opening statements, and I will be very brief because I don't have that much to say about it, my children think I remember that 1918 Spanish Flu pandemic, but I do remember and was affected by it because I knew people that had lost children during that time. And when you lose three-quarters of a million people in this country at a day and time when we didn't have that many people in this country, that was quite a loss and quite a huge percentage of people that were affected by it.

I have said here and as I hear this I thought of a hearing I held in the Science Committee some 4, 5, or 6 years ago on asteroids. And we were all surprised to find out that an asteroid had just missed the United States by about 15 minutes in 1988, one the size of maybe Delaware or one of the other States. We were a little surprised at that. We might also have some surprises when we hear your testimony, because we don't know by how much we have missed epidemics and what has been done about it.

But I think we are very fortunate to have learned people like you with your years of study and your research on vaccines and for things to do for it, that you have prepared yourself for prevention, and if not prevention, control. I thank you for giving your time and I think that it is a timely thing that we need to hear and need to know more about. Mr. Chairman, I thank you for having it. I yield back my time.

Mr. DEAL. I thank the gentleman. Recognize the gentleman from California, Mr. Waxman, for an opening statement.

Mr. WAXMAN. Mr. Chairman, I thank you for calling this hearing today and drawing attention to this very important issue. Many leading scientists believe that it is not a matter of if but when the next flu pandemic will hit. It has been estimated that even a medium-level pandemic could cause up to 200,000 deaths in the United States and 734,000 hospitalizations at a cost of up to $166 billion. Pandemic flu is a grave public health threat, and we must do all we can to get ready for it.

There are many unknowns surrounding the pandemic flu. It is unknown which strain of the flu virus would cause the pandemic, so production of an effective vaccine must wait until the pandemic begins. It is unknown how long it will take to produce a vaccine. It is also an unknown whether or how well antiviral medications will work. With so many unknowns it is easy to become very anxious about this topic. Fortunately, there are some things we do know, and these are some steps we can take now to be prepared no matter what the strain of the pandemic virus, no matter how long it takes to make a vaccine, no matter how well antiviral medications work, our core public health system must be strong. We must have a way to deliver vaccines to those most at risk quickly and efficiently.

This year's flu shortage illustrated how far away we are from this capability. Many chronically ill and elderly Americans were forced to wait for hours just to get their vaccines. We must do better than this. We also must have the ability to maintain core public health functions in the event of a pandemic. One major vaccine manufacturer has told us that in order to produce the necessary vaccines to combat a flu pandemic, the company would have to dramatically curtail production of its childhood vaccines. This would be a particularly dangerous situation given that stockpiles of many childhood vaccines do not exist. It would be a disaster if our preparation for flu pandemic led to outbreak of childhood diseases. But that could happen.

That is why today we must do more than ask our expert witnesses to speculate about uncertainties. We must also ask some tough questions about the administration's response to the challenges as plain as day. We also must ask why the administration has proposed major cuts in funding for key programs in State and local preparedness. These are the very programs that allow our communities to prepare for bioterrorism, natural disasters, and a flu pandemic. We must also ask why the administration has yet again failed to provide adequate funding for States for vaccines against preventable diseases. If we cannot even stop bacterial meningitis from spreading in our communities even when we have vaccines, how will we stop the flu virus? And we must ask why it has taken so long to get senior administration officials to focus their attention on lack of stockpiles for routine pediatric illness. These stockpiles were promised 3 years ago, and yet a letter asking about the holdup was sent to vaccine manufacturers just 2 days ago.

After we ask these tough questions it will be time to get back to work, and I hope we can join together across party lines to support major improvements in our public health system. I thank the witnesses for attending and look forward to their testimony.

Mr. DEAL. Recognize the gentlelady from California, Ms. Bono, for opening statement.

Ms. BONO. Thank you, Mr. Chairman. I will waive my opening statement.

Mr. DEAL. Recognize Mr. Green from Texas for an opening statement.

Mr. GREEN. Thank you, Mr. Chairman, and thank you and the ranking member for holding the hearing on the threat of pandemic flu and the steps we are taking to protect Americans from the outbreak. Hopefully, we will get ahead of the curve. I also want to thank our panelists this morning who—as a lot of us feel like—listen to us give our statements, but oftentimes it is the only time members on the committee can do anything except vote.

I have a personal interest in this issue because my daughter has been accepted in a medical fellowship on infectious diseases, and so I am particularly thankful that I can gain some knowledge in one of the issues that she certainly is working with now in the forefront of her medical work. I tell her I don't want to be treated for anything she studies.

The 20th century was a witness to three flu pandemics, so we know what kind of destruction these outbreaks can cause. And recent press reports suggest we are dangerously close to witnessing another. According to the World Health Organization, the next pandemic flu would likely result in 1 to 2.3 million hospitalizations and 300 to 650,000 deaths in developed countries alone. We can only imagine the kind of havoc that a pandemic flu would wreak on developing nations which do not have the healthcare infrastructure surveillance capabilities to protect their citizens from infectious disease.

Where I ought to know this is to be the case is poor countries facing the threat of the Bird Flu since the current outbreak in 2003 have been unable to successfully detect and respond to individual cases of Bird Flu. The influenza strain that most concerns infectious disease specialists is the H5N1 strain has jumped from animals to human and to date has killed 36 people in Vietnam, 12 in Thailand, and four in Cambodia. And while the Bird Flu has thus far been contained in Asia, the WHO influenza specialists recognize this can't last that long with the amount of contact we have literally in our very small world now.

We know that human flu pandemic will consist of three elements in tandem. The Bird Flu has already presented us with a virus to which humans have little or no immunity. The deaths in Asia have proven that this virus can replicate itself in humans causing serious illness, if not death. The virus may also be transmittable from human to human. Since this current outbreak in 2003, the third element has not been met. However, Dr. Fauci's testimony today indicates a high probability where they not have witnessed at least once case of human-to-human transmission in H5N1 virus. Given this news, the hearing is particularly timely. The subcommittee has held hearings in the past about our supply of flu vaccine in this country and the challenges that face both the government and the vaccine manufacturers. This hearing, I hope, will build on previous knowledge we gained from our subcommittee's activities and shed light on steps we must take to ensure an adequate and effective vaccine supply to protect Americans from the deadly flu pandemic.

And, again, I would like to thank our witnesses for being here and for what you do every day to protect our constituents. Thank you, Mr. Chairman.

Mr. DEAL. I thank the gentleman. We are ready now for our first panel and—well, I have another member. Mr. Pitts, do you wish to make an opening statement? All right. You have already heard everything that we know about this issue. Now we are looking forward to hearing what you know about it. I would remind you we have your written testimony, which is a part of the record. And, Dr. Gerberding, we will start with you.

STATEMENTS OF JULIE L. GERBERDING, DIRECTOR, CENTERS FOR DISEASE CONTROL AND PREVENTION, DEPARTMENT OF HEALTH AND HUMAN SERVICES; ANTHONY S. FAUCI, DIRECTOR, NATIONAL INSTITUTE OF ALLERGY AND INFECTIOUS DISEASES, NATIONAL INSTITUTES OF HEALTH, DEPARTMENT OF HEALTH AND HUMAN SERVICES; AND BRUCE G. GELLIN, DIRECTOR, NATIONAL VACCINE PROGRAM OFFICE, DEPARTMENT OF HEALTH AND HUMAN SERVICES

Ms. GERBERDING. Thank you. I am absolutely grateful to the committee for having this hearing. I think the more we shine a bright light on this problem, the more we will be able to be prepared to handle it. Your eloquence in describing both the severity of the threat as well as the impact is heartening. And I think I speak for all of us in the Department of Health and Human Services and Secretary Leavitt, we know this is a high priority for the agency. Secretary Leavitt has been meeting with us almost every day on flu since he took office. And at the World Health Assembly last week where all of the leaders of the health community around the globe assembled in Geneva, the secretary convened several discussions on influenza pandemic planning and how we could assist.

What I am going to try to do today is two things in my brief remarks: one is just give a capsule situation report on the flu in Asia, and second, describe in brief some of the important steps that we are already taking. We are not waiting for that final preparedness plan to get approved. We are acting now to get the show on the road.

Just as a reminder for those who aren't familiar with influenza, you will be hearing us talking about H5N1 or H3N2. Flu is a simple little virus with just a few genes. One of them codes for something called "H" or hemagglutinin and the other codes for "N", neuraminidase. But despite its simplicity, this is a very sinister virus, and it changes all the time. When the changes in H and N are little or small in genetic context, it is called a drift, and that is what happens every year and why we need to get a new flu shot every year. Sometimes we see a shift, which is a major change. Usually the virus exchanges genes with some other strain of flu and you see a big jump in the composition in the H or the N, and that is the change that is usually associated with pandemics.

[Chart]

Ms. GERBERDING. This is a map of the prior influenza pandemics that have occurred throughout the last 100 years, and you can see that each time there is a big shift in the H gene from H1 to H2; the Asian Flu appeared when H2 came on the horizon. When H3 appeared we saw the Hong Kong Flu pandemic.

And what you are seeing in upper corner here are H7, H5, and H9, which are Avian isolates not yet transmitted in broad scale to people in pandemics, but certainly on the horizon and very ominous because we, of course, have no population immunity to any of those H's. And so because we are seeing right now H5 and 1 in Asia, we are particularly concerned about the emergence of the virus in a world that has absolutely no immunity.

How do these big jumps occur? Well, it is a complicated story, but often what happens is that a virus from a bird host—in this case an asymptomatic duck, or in Asia right now, the poultry that are infected—can commingle in a pig usually with a human virus and exchange those big genes resulting in a completely new virus that then gets transmitted to people. But in this context in Asia today, we are also concerned about the direct transfer of the poultry virus to humans. And this, we know, has occurred a number of times.

The reason this is so critical and why we are focusing so much on Asia is that in China alone there are 1.3 billion people, but there are 13 billion chickens and about 508 million pigs. So in that area of the world if you multiply that by the incredible density of population, we are sitting on the cauldron of flu virus incubation, and the threat is certainly one that we are taking very seriously.

These are the numbers of people so far who have been reported to the World Health Organization with this H5N1 Avian Flu: 97 people in total with a fatality rate of 55 percent. This may be the tip of the iceberg; we don't know. But it certainly is a cause of concern. And recently there has been some suggestion of more clustering in at least one region of Vietnam and perhaps the suggestion that the virus is slowly becoming more adaptable to humans. Of course, that remains to be seen.

This map shows some of the indicators of poultry virus activity in this region. I have occluded status: unknown here as China because just this week we learned about the migratory bird die-off in Western China, which was related to a species of geese called the Bar-headed Goose that migrates up from India and the Tibetan Plateau, and a reliable laboratory in China has indicated that that indeed was H5N1 virus.

So we are seeing mass populations of poultry throughout Asia infected. And all of the activities that we are doing right now at HHS are targeting, first and foremost, preparedness in that region. We are very pleased with the recent supplemental appropriation from Congress for CDC and USAID to receive $25 million to step up activities in Asia and another $58 million to augment our supplies in preparation for the stockpile.

But we are doing a lot of other things at CDC and HHS as well. We are utilizing all of our laboratory networks, we are developing rapid diagnostic tests, we are working on expanding our capacity for vaccine seed development, our virus genomic activities to characterize these strains and their drug susceptibility, and certainly Dr. Fauci will talk about how all that feeds into vaccine development.

Last, just let me mention that this map of the various teams of people at CDC is just a microcosm of what is gong on throughout HHS and the entire public health system. We are working with all sectors, including public health, healthcare, business, and communications experts, but we are also taking advantage of the $287 million in appropriation that we did receive this year to support flu activities in our agency. Those appropriations are being used to purchase influenza vaccine, to purchase antivirals for influenza from the department, to support improvements in the vaccine manufacturing and science, as well as many other investments to help speed and accelerate our preparedness for this very uncertain virus.

So we look forward to answering specific questions about the steps that we are taking, the preparedness, but I wanted to assure that, again, we are not waiting for a written plan; we are acting now to do everything we can with the resources that we do have. And we are particularly focusing those resources on Asia where we feel the imminence of the situation is probably deserving of our greatest attention. Thank you.

[The prepared statement of Julie L. Gerberding follows:]

PREPARED STATEMENT OF JULIE L. GERBERDING, DIRECTOR, CENTERS FOR DISEASE CONTROL AND PREVENTION, U.S. DEPARTMENT OF HEALTH AND HUMAN SERVICES

Mr. Chairman and members of the Subcommittee, I am pleased to be here today to describe planning and preparedness for an influenza pandemic, including the potential threat posed by the H5N1 avian influenza virus currently in Asia. Department of Health and Human Services Secretary Mike Leavitt has made influenza pandemic planning and preparedness one of his top priorities; and each agency within the Department is working together to prepare the United States for a potential threat to the health of our nation.

I will discuss steps the Centers for Disease Control and Prevention (CDC) is taking with many partners both domestically and globally. The strength and flexibility of CDC and other components of the public health system are vital assets as the United States sharpens its readiness for an influenza pandemic. Although we have made significant progress, more work is needed, particularly in the areas of surveillance capacity and response, and the development of potential vaccines. Increased public awareness and understanding about infection control, containment, and other actions also are important in preparation for an influenza pandemic.

PANDEMICS IN PERSPECTIVE

Seasonal influenza causes an average of 36,000 deaths each year in the United States, mostly among the elderly and nearly 200,000 hospitalizations. In contrast, the actual severity and impact of the next pandemic, whether from H5N1 or another influenza virus, cannot be predicted. However, modeling studies suggest that, in the absence of any control measures, such as vaccination, a "medium-level" pandemic in the United States could result in 89,000 to 207,000 deaths, between 314,000 and 734,000 hospitalizations, 18 to 42 million outpatient visits, and another 20 to 47 million people being sick. Between 15 percent and 35 percent of the United States population could be affected by an influenza pandemic, and the economic impact in our country alone could range between $71.3 and $166.5 billion.

A public health response to a disease of this magnitude involves numerous challenges.

- A pandemic can occur any time during the year and can last much longer than seasonal influenza.
- In more advanced pandemic phases, the capacity to prevent or control transmission of the virus can become extremely difficult.
- Although the primary concern at present is the H5N1 avian influenza strain in Asia, an outbreak leading to a pandemic can occur anywhere in the world and may derive from viral strains of influenza other than H5N1.
- Comparing the onset and spread of the next pandemic to those of the 20th century is problematic for many reasons, including changes in population and social structures, medical and technological advances, and the increase in international travel.
- With zoonotic diseases such as avian influenza, there is a need for coordination with the animal health community.

THE CURRENT SITUATION IN ASIA

For an influenza virus to cause a pandemic, it must meet three major criteria: (1) possess a new surface protein to which there is little or no pre-existing immunity in the human population; (2) be able to cause illness in humans; and (3) have the ability for *sustained* transmission from person to person. So far, the H5N1 virus has met two of these three criteria, but it has not yet shown the capability for sustained transmission from person to person.

Concerning this third point, it is important to keep in mind the close relationship of viral infections in animal hosts and those in humans. Ongoing dialogue between agricultural and public health officials is extremely important for the careful, consistent surveillance necessary in both animal and human populations. Although the present avian influenza H5N1 strain in Asia does not yet have the capability of sustained person-to-person transmission, chicken-to-human transmission has occurred, and in at least one cluster, limited person-to-person transmission has been identified. As of May 19, 2005 the World Health Organization (WHO) had confirmed 97 cases of H5N1 influenza in humans since January 28, 2004, with a case fatality rate of 55 percent. The World Organization for Animal Health (OIE) confirmed, as of May 13, 2005, that H5N1 had been found in animals from nine Asian countries in 2004 and 2005, with especially large outbreaks among animals in Vietnam and Thailand. Millions of domestic birds have been culled in attempts to stop the spread of the virus among animal populations.

Although human case fatality rates seem to have gone down somewhat since February 2005, CDC, WHO, and other partners are still quite concerned for several reasons. The H5N1 strain now appears to be endemic in poultry and other birds in a number of Asian countries, signaling a potential long-term threat of mutation and reassortment with other viral strains. Recent studies have found that ducks carry the H5N1 strain asymptomatically, making it difficult to monitor the magnitude of transmission from ducks to other species. Confirmation that H5N1 also has been transmitted to mammals is a particular concern, because of the increased potential of the strain to reassort with other strains already common to humans and other mammals. Studies have documented highly pathogenic H5N1 in pigs, tigers, and leopards in Asia. Difficulties in implementing effective in-country surveillance, including enhancing the training of laboratorians, epidemiologists, veterinarians, and other professionals, inhibit the type of comprehensive reporting that is essential to monitor H5N1 and other strains of highly pathogenic avian influenza. Finally, changes in the epidemiology of the infections, such as decreasing mortality rates, could indicate changes that make the viruses better adapted to humans. Additional studies and research are needed to better understand the current situation and how the viruses may be changing.

RESPONDING TO A PANDEMIC

An effective response to an influenza pandemic requires highly collaborative planning, implementation, and flexibility in resolving issues at many levels. The Department of Health and Human Services (DHHS) is leading the coordination of preparedness efforts through its *Pandemic Influenza Response and Preparedness Plan,* which was released in draft form in August 2004 for public comment and is under revision. In addition, states are either developing pandemic influenza plans or revising existing plans to reflect new information and data. Key elements of these plans include surveillance, infection control, use of antiviral medications, community containment measures, vaccination procedures, communications, and ability to sustain essential services in times of widespread illness. Similar elements inform a plan that CDC is developing, that will provide detailed guidance and materials to states and localities and will complement the DHHS plan. CDC also will take the lead in working with the Advisory Committee on Immunization Practices and the National Vaccine Advisory Committee to prioritize recommended target groups for use of antiviral medications and vaccines during a pandemic when supplies are limited.

Once a pandemic strain starts circulating in the United States, isolation precautions for persons who are ill and quarantine for persons exposed may need to be considered to limit the early spread of pandemic influenza, particularly before a vaccine becomes available. Measures such as these will require a multi-level, multi-faceted, staged process, such as evaluating all ill travelers arriving from affected areas. On April 1, 2005 the President amended Executive Order 13295, adding influenza caused by novel or reemergent influenza viruses that are causing, or have the potential to cause, a pandemic to the list of quarantinable diseases. CDC has implemented a series of travel notices to minimize the potential for outbreaks to extend to wider geographic areas. CDC also has expanded the number and capacity of its quarantine stations at major ports of entry into the United States. As with any quarantine, such activities need to be undertaken judiciously to minimize adverse impacts on civil liberties.

Vaccination is the best long-term strategy for influenza prevention and control, both during annual outbreaks and a pandemic; antiviral medications provide an earlier, secondary line of defense. Other measures may help control the spread of influenza in a pandemic situation, such as isolation of ill persons and quarantine of healthy exposed persons. Comprehensive preparedness for annual influenza outbreaks is a vital component of an effective response to pandemic influenza, although pandemic planning will require additional preparation activities.

SURVEILLANCE

The United States, working domestically and with global partners, needs to expand the scope of early-warning surveillance activities used to detect the next pandemic. We cannot estimate the amount of time from first detection in another country to peak disease in the United States, but it could be a matter of months or less. Time will be of the essence in making sure we can produce, test, and administer vaccine as quickly as possible. It will take several months for the first dose of pandemic vaccine to be ready and longer to manufacture enough to vaccinate the entire U.S. population. Therefore, vaccine will be in short supply at the start of the pandemic. Under the most favorable conditions, by the time the first dose of vaccine would be given to the first person, many others will have already become ill or died. For this reason, surveillance to monitor ongoing changes in the H5N1 strain of avian influenza currently causing human infections and to monitor for other viruses with pandemic potential is needed to develop prototype vaccine candidates as quickly as possible. Further, because such a pandemic strain can arise anywhere, at any time, expanded global surveillance capacity is needed.

The outbreaks of avian influenza in Asia have highlighted several gaps in disease surveillance globally that the United States must help address to improve our ability to prepare for an influenza pandemic. These challenges include: (1) lack of infrastructure in many countries for in-country surveillance networks; (2) need for increased training of laboratory, epidemiologic, and veterinary staff; and (3) resolution of longstanding obstacles to rapid and open sharing of surveillance information, specimens, and viruses among agriculture and human health authorities in affected countries and the international community. CDC and HHS have made significant progress in the past year toward enhancing surveillance in Southeast Asia. This initiative needs to continue at both national and international levels if we are to expand geographic coverage and develop an adequate capacity to conduct effective surveillance. These efforts, in turn, will increase our ability to detect new variants earlier, make more informed vaccine decisions for yearly epidemics, and build an "early warning system" for new viruses that may cause a pandemic. With the ever-present threat of the emergence of a new pandemic strain, we need to know what is happening in the backyards of Southeast Asia, as well as elsewhere throughout the world. Year-round, world-wide surveillance for infections of humans with new strains of influenza is essential for us to prepare for the next pandemic, as well as for next year's epidemic. Recently, the Congress passed and the President signed an FY 2005 Emergency Supplemental Appropriations Act for Defense, the Global War on Terror, and Tsunami Relief, which included $25 million in international assistance funds to prevent and control the spread of avian influenza in Southeast Asia. These funds will support human surveillance, laboratory capacity, and enhanced knowledge of state-of-the-art avian influenza laboratory and field techniques in Southeast Asia.

In the past year, CDC has considerably improved domestic surveillance, adding two new major components to our surveillance system. We worked with the Council for State and Territorial Epidemiologists (CSTE) to make confirmed pediatric deaths from influenza nationally notifiable, and we implemented hospital-based surveillance for influenza in children at selected sites. To further improve our understanding of the impact of influenza on severe outcomes, such as hospitalization, we are working with the CSTE to make all laboratory confirmed influenza hospitalizations notifiable. We have issued interim guidelines to states and hospitals to enhance surveillance for potential cases of people infected by avian influenza on several occasions and these enhancements continue. CDC also set up special laboratory training courses for identification of avian influenza using rapid molecular techniques. So far, professionals from 48 states and Washington D.C. have been trained.

However, to be as prepared as possible for a pandemic, we are working to do much more in the domestic surveillance arena. The United States is working to: (1) ensure that states have sufficient epidemiologic and laboratory capacity both to identify novel viruses throughout the year and to sustain surveillance during a pandemic; (2) improve reporting systems so that information needed to make public health decisions is available quickly; (3) enhance systems for identifying and reporting severe cases of influenza; (4) develop population-based surveillance among adults hospitalized with influenza and (5) enhance monitoring of resistance to current antiviral drugs, to guide policy for use of scarce antiviral drugs.

MANAGING THE VACCINE SUPPLY

During an influenza pandemic, the presence of U.S.-based manufacturing facilities will be critically important. The pandemic influenza vaccines produced in other countries will likely not be available to the US market as those governments may prohibit export of the vaccines produced in their countries until their domestic needs are met. However, the vaccine manufacturing system in the United States is fragile. Currently, there are only three influenza vaccine manufacturers producing vaccines for the US market, and only one produces its vaccine entirely in the United States.

During the past several years, CDC and other DHHS agencies have developed several new strategies to address annual influenza outbreaks, including the support of enhanced vaccine production, and have worked to ensure a better match of vaccine distribution to the populations in greatest need. Public demand for influenza vaccine on a yearly basis needs to be both stabilized and increased, so that companies will have a growing market to provide an incentive to increase production. These strategies include $40 million for purchasing influenza vaccine for the pediatric stockpile to protect against annual outbreaks of influenza, and $30 million will be used for contracts to expand the production of bulk single-strain influenza vaccine for use if needed during annual influenza season or possibly in a pandemic situation. In addition, the President is requesting $120—million in fiscal year 2006, an increase of $21 million, to encourage greater production capacity that will enhance the U.S.-based vaccine manufacturing surge capacity to help prepare for a pandemic and further guard against annual shortages.

The Department also appreciates the inclusion of $58 million in the FY 2005 Emergency Supplemental to procure additional influenza countermeasures for the CDC Strategic National Stockpile (SNS) in FY 2005. Currently, the SNS has enough oseltamivir (Tamiflu) capsules to treat approximately 2.26 million adults and oseltamivir (Tamiflu) suspension to treat more than 100,000 children. In addition, SNS contains enough rimantadine tablets to treat up to 4.25 million people and enough rimantadine suspension to treat up to 750,000. It should be noted, however, that oseltamivir is the only antiviral at this time shown to be effective against the H5N1 avian influenza virus in Asia. In addition, SNS funds have been used to purchase approximately 2 million bulk doses of unfinished, unfilled H5N1 vaccine, although it is not yet formulated into vials nor is the vaccine licensed. Clinical testing to determine dosage and schedule for this vaccine began in April 2005 with funding from the National Institutes of Health.

DHHS also is supporting the development and testing of potential dose-sparing strategies to extend a given quantity of vaccine stock.

Regarding annual influenza vaccination, there is an emerging consensus that it is desirable to expand vaccine coverage beyond the high priority groups for whom routine vaccination is already recommended. Discussions are under way to review the data that would be needed to consider broadening recommendations for influenza vaccination. CDC is developing strategies to increase informed demand for, and access to, influenza vaccine for persons who are currently recommended to be vaccinated each year. For example, according to a 2003 Institute of Medicine report, an estimated 8.2 million additional high-risk uninsured adults 18-64 years old warrant annual vaccination. We recognize that these at-risk persons need better access to vaccine during a pandemic as well as for seasonal influenza.

Additionally, CDC, in conjunction with the Advisory Committee on Immunization Practices, is developing an internal set of possible influenza vaccine supply scenarios that may occur in future influenza seasons and during a pandemic. These scenarios range from worst-case to best-case situations and are an important part of CDC planning efforts. We are preparing recommendations, plans, and communication messages for any of the possible situations.

CONCLUSION

Although the present avian influenza H5N1 strain in Southeast Asia does not yet have the capability of sustained person-to-person transmission, we are concerned that it could. CDC is closely monitoring the situation in collaboration with the World Health Organization. CDC is using its extensive network of partnerships with other federal agencies, provider groups, non-profit organizations, vaccine and antiviral manufacturers, and state and local health departments to enhance pandemic influenza planning. Our responses to the annual domestic influenza seasons also will inform the nation's planning and preparedness for pandemic influenza. The same laboratories, health care providers, surveillance systems, and health department plans and personnel guide both responses. These actions, in conjunction with increased public understanding about influenza, will help us all prepare for an influenza pandemic.

Thank you for this opportunity to share this information with you. I am happy to answer any questions.

Mr. DEAL. Thank you. Dr. Fauci.

STATEMENT OF ANTHONY S. FAUCI

Mr. FAUCI. Thank you very much, Mr. Chairman, and thank you for giving me the opportunity to address this committee on the research component of the department's effort in preparedness against pandemic flu.

[Slide]

Mr. FAUCI. I would like to put this into perspective by showing you first this initial slide, which shows the complimentary roles of the sister agencies within HHS regarding how we approach pandemic flu preparedness. Dr. Gerberding has explained to you the CDC's role. The FDA plays an important regulatory role, particularly with regard to the countermeasure that are used, both therapeutics and vaccines. I am going to spend my couple of minutes describing for you some of the research endeavors that range from fundamental basic science up through and including the development of countermeasures. All of this, of course, is coordinated under the office of Public Health Emergency Preparedness at the department.

This slide illustrates the multifaceted component of the research endeavor. You see on the lower-left we refer to a surveillance and epidemiology, which is really fundamentally the CDC's role. We play a very small role in that, and that is at the molecular level to try and characterize the evolving, changing viruses, particularly those that occur in animal species, as just described by Dr. Gerberding.

In addition, we train and provide both physical and intellectual capacity and, importantly, the basic research understanding of the virus and how it works helps us in our endeavor to make vaccines, therapeutics, and diagnostics.

I am going to spend just a moment describing two examples of some of the basic approaches toward influenza which have helped us in the development of vaccines. Some of you may have heard of the terminology "reverse genetics." What that is is a molecular sophisticated way to take away some of the uncertainty of providing that seed virus that you need to make a vaccine. What it does is deliberately take the genes from a virus that we know grows very well in our egg cultures and then ultimately, hopefully, some day in cell-based cultures, as well as the important genes from the index virus in question—in this case it is an H5N1—and deliberately put them together to predictably get the seed virus that will be used for the vaccine. And in fact this is just what we did with the H5N1 that is currently in clinical trials, as I will describe to you in a moment.

Another research endeavor is that which we are doing in collaboration with the CDC and industry is to provide a consistent way to get cell-based cultures to ultimately transition and replace the egg-based cultures. And the reason for that is that the surge capacity of having the ability to grow cells in culture all year round so that if you either have to change direction or surge up in numbers, that system is much more adaptable than the egg-based system, which has its very good, positive points.

Having said all of this, and I hope we get into the discussion, that despite the effort, despite the research, the capacity globally to make vaccines for H5N1, as several of the members have alluded to, is really one of the great limiting issues that we have to face, and I hope we get back to that.

Let me just spend a moment talking about the influenza vaccine trials. Dr. Gerberding mentioned and I want to underscore that we are not waiting for anything to move ahead to address this problem. We have an H5N1 from Vietnam and we have a trial that has already yielded data. There are two major trials. The inactivated vaccine trial began on April 4, 2005 in three medical centers in the United States. It is in multiple stages involving four doses, a prime initial vaccine, followed by a boost. The reason we have to do that when we don't generally have to do that with the seasonal vaccine that we change a bit every year is that our population, or the population of the world, has never experienced an H5N1. So we don't really know what the proper dose is or whether or not we are going to need, and we likely will need, a prime and a boost. So we have divided the trial into stages. We fully enrolled the first 118 adults in Stage 1; we fully enrolled the second stage for a total of 450. By early to mid-summer we will have safety data and data about how to use that, what is the right dose, and then we will move onto the elderly—greater than 65—and then we will go to children.

There is also an H9N2 trial going as well as attenuated vaccine trials. So there are multiple things going ahead, and we are clearly ahead of any other country in the trial of the relevant H5N1 right now.

Again, just a word on antiviral therapy. We know that H5N1 is sensitive to oseltamivir and relatively resistant to the other class of drugs. We are doing research both in understanding how best to use the existing drugs alone or in combination in adults and in children, as well as targeting other targets of the influenza replication cycle so that we will have a pipeline of drugs should resistance emerge.

And finally, just to recapitulate and underscore that the NIH research effort is fundamentally based on basic research but is rapidly applying that to the development of countermeasures, particularly in the form of vaccines and therapeutics that will be part of the broad Department of Health and Human Services Pandemic Preparedness Plan. I would be happy to answer your questions later. Thank you very much, Mr. Chairman.

[The prepared statement of Anthony S. Fauci follows:]

PREPARED STATEMENT OF ANTHONY S. FAUCI, DIRECTOR, NATIONAL INSTITUTE OF ALLERGY AND INFECTIOUS DISEASES, NATIONAL INSTITUTES OF HEALTH, DEPARTMENT OF HEALTH AND HUMAN SERVICES

INTRODUCTION

Mr. Chairman and Members of the Committee, thank you for the opportunity to discuss with you the role of the National Institutes of Health (NIH) in preparing the Nation for the next influenza pandemic. The Department of Health and Human Services (DHHS) Draft Pandemic Influenza Preparedness and Response Plan outlines a coordinated national strategy to prepare for and respond to an influenza pandemic, and assigns specific roles to various Federal agencies; the National Institute of Allergy and Infectious Diseases (NIAID) holds the primary responsibility for carrying out those duties assigned to NIH.

In this capacity, NIAID provides the scientific input required to facilitate the development of both new influenza vaccine technologies and novel antiviral drugs against influenza viruses. Under this Administration, we have made extraordinary progress. DHHS began investing in new technologies, securing more vaccines and medicines, and preparing stronger response plans. Total NIH funding for influenza research has grown more than five-fold in recent years, from $20.6 million in FY 2001 to an estimated $119 million in FY 2005. This is part of the largest investment ever made by the Federal government in protecting against influenza.

Influenza epidemics typically occur during the winter months in the United States and other temperate regions of the world and cause significant morbidity and mortality. On average, 36,000 people in this country die each year and 200,000 are hospitalized due to influenza and influenza-related complications. Each year, influenza viruses undergo small changes in their surface proteins as they circulate through the human population. As these small changes accumulate, the influenza virus gains the ability to overcome immunity created by prior exposure to older circulating influenza viruses or by vaccination. This phenomenon, called "antigenic drift," is the basis for the well-recognized patterns of influenza disease that occur every year, and is the reason that influenza vaccines must be updated each year.

Influenza viruses can also change more dramatically; viruses may emerge that can jump species from natural reservoirs such as wild ducks to infect domestic poultry, farm animals, or humans. This type of significant change in the antigenic make-up of the virus that infects humans is referred to as "antigenic shift."

In most instances when influenza virus jumps species from an animal such as a chicken to infect a human, the result is a "dead end" infection that cannot readily be transmitted further from human to human. Mutations in the virus, however, could increase the efficiency of human-to-human transmission. Furthermore, if an avian influenza virus and another human influenza virus were to simultaneously co-infect a person, the genes of the two viruses might reassort, resulting in a virus that is readily transmissible between humans and against which the population would have no natural immunity. In addition, the reassortant virus could reflect the virulence of the avian virus. Such a virus could potentially cause an influenza pandemic.

Historically, pandemic influenza is a proven threat. Three influenza pandemics have occurred in the 20th century: in 1918, 1957, and 1968. The 1918-1919 pandemic was by far the most severe, killing approximately 500,000 people in the United States and 20-40 million people worldwide—almost two percent of the global population at that time. Worldwide, the pandemics that began in 1957 and 1968 killed approximately 2 million and 700,000 people, respectively.

H9N2 and H5N1 influenza are two avian viruses that have jumped directly from birds to humans and have significant pandemic potential. In 1999 and 2003, H9N2 influenza caused illness in three people in Hong Kong and in five individuals elsewhere in China, but the virus did not spread from human to human. H5N1 influenza, often referred to as "bird flu," appears to be a significantly greater threat than

H9N2. This virus was first detected in humans in Hong Kong in 1997. Since January 2004, it has spread widely among wild and domestic birds and has infected at least 97 people in Vietnam, Thailand, and Cambodia; 53 of these people have died of the disease. Ominously, H5N1 viruses are evolving in ways that increasingly favor the start of a pandemic, including becoming more stable in the environment and expanding their host species range. Moreover, there has been at least one highly probable case of human-to-human transmission of the H5N1 virus, and it is possible that other such transmissions have occurred recently.

The deadly experience with past influenza pandemics explains our current high level of concern about the appearance of virulent H5N1 avian influenza viruses in Asia, which by a variety of mechanisms could adapt themselves to efficiently spread from human to human and result in the next pandemic. Given the poor condition of public health systems in many underdeveloped regions and the speed of modern air travel, the consequences of such an event, should it result in an influenza pandemic, would be severe.

NIH INFLUENZA RESEARCH ACTIVITIES

Between influenza pandemics, when influenza activity occurs regularly on a seasonal basis, the role of NIAID is to conduct basic research into the viral biology, pathogenesis, and epidemiology of influenza viruses and to study host immune responses to these agents. Concomitant with these basic research studies, NIAID conducts applied research to develop new or improved influenza vaccines and production methods; to identify new anti-influenza drugs; and to support surveillance for previously unknown influenza viruses in animals and characterize any that are found. When a new influenza virus begins to infect humans (and thereby gains the potential to cause a pandemic), NIAID's role is to develop and clinically evaluate specific candidate vaccines against the emergent strain, test the activity of antiviral drugs, and, in some cases, supply vaccine manufacturers and the research community with viral reference strains and other reagents to speed vaccine development.

BASIC RESEARCH

NIAID supports many basic research projects intended to increase our understanding of how influenza viruses replicate, interact with their hosts, stimulate immune responses, and evolve into new strains. Results from these studies lay the foundation for the design of new antiviral drugs, diagnostics, and vaccines, and are applicable to seasonal epidemic and pandemic strains alike.

NIAID also supports two special research programs to better understand the diversity of influenza viruses. The Influenza Genome Sequencing Project, launched in the fall of 2004, is a collaboration between NIAID, the Centers for Disease Control and Prevention (CDC) and several other organizations to determine the complete genetic sequences of thousands of influenza virus isolates and to rapidly provide these sequence data to the scientific community. This program will enable scientists to better understand the emergence of influenza epidemics and pandemics by observing how influenza viruses evolve as they spread through the population and by matching viral genetic characteristics with virulence, ease of transmissibility, and other properties. As of May 24, 2005, 182 genomic sequences of influenza viruses had been made available through this program to researchers via the NIH website, and many more are in the pipeline.

NIAID also supports a long-standing program based in Hong Kong to detect the emergence of influenza viruses with pandemic potential. This program, led by Dr. Robert Webster of St. Jude Children's Research Hospital in Memphis, Tennessee, conducts extensive surveillance of influenza viruses in animals in Hong Kong, analyzes new influenza viruses when they are found, and helps to generate candidate vaccines against them. In January, the scope of this surveillance program was expanded to include Vietnam, Thailand, and Indonesia.

Vaccines

Vaccines are essential tools for the control of influenza. NIAID supports numerous research projects and other initiatives to foster the development of new influenza vaccine candidates and manufacturing methods that are simpler, more reliable, yield more broadly cross-protective products, and provide alternatives to the egg-based technology currently used to grow the vaccine viruses.

In the Fiscal Year 2006 budget request, DHHS has requested $120 million to support pandemic influenza preparedness activities. These activities build on previous initiatives that include making chicken eggs available year round to provide for a secure supply and surge capacity for vaccine production and supporting efforts to shift vaccine manufacture to new cell-culture technologies. Moreover, a technique developed by NIAID-supported scientists called reverse genetics allows scientists to manipulate the genomes of influenza viruses and to transfer genes between viral strains. This technique allows the rapid generation of vaccine candidate strains that precisely match a selected epidemic strain. By removing or modifying certain virulence genes, reverse genetics also can be used to convert highly pathogenic influenza viruses into vaccine candidates that are safer for vaccine manufacturers to handle. Other vaccine strategies for influenza, including protein subunit and gene-based vaccines, are also being actively pursued. On the NIH campus in Bethesda, the NIAID Vaccine Research Center (VRC) has initiated a program to develop gene-based vaccines against influenza. Should proof-of-concept studies prove successful, the VRC expects to expand and accelerate the development of gene-based and recombinant influenza vaccines.

In addition to supporting the development of new vaccine strategies, NIAID maintains an extensive capacity for evaluating candidate vaccines in clinical trials. For example, NIAID's Vaccine and Treatment Evaluation Units (VTEUs) comprise a network of university-based research medical centers across the United States that conduct clinical trials to test candidate vaccines for many infectious diseases. These units support both academic and industrial vaccine evaluation, including safety, immunogenicity, and ultimately, efficacy of candidate vaccines.

Although a pandemic alert has not yet been declared, NIAID has taken a number of steps to develop and clinically test vaccines against H5N1 and H9N2 influenza, two specific avian viruses that have significant pandemic potential. For example, in August 2004, NIAID contracted with Chiron Corporation for the production of 40,000 doses of an inactivated H9N2 vaccine. A Phase I clinical trial of this vaccine began on March 31, 2005, and is fully enrolled.

In January 2004, researchers at St. Jude Children's Research Hospital obtained a clinical isolate of the highly virulent H5N1 virus that was fatal to humans in Vietnam in late 2003 and early 2004 and used reverse genetics to create an H5N1 candidate vaccine from this strain. Immediately after NIAID received this vaccine last June, it was sent to two companies, Sanofi-Pasteur (formerly Aventis-Pasteur) and Chiron, which have NIAID contracts to manufacture pilot lots of eight and ten thousand vaccine doses, respectively. The vaccines will be tested in Phase I and II clinical trials that will assess safety and the appropriate dose to optimize immunogenicity, as well as provide information about how the immune system responds to this vaccine. The Sanofi-Pasteur trial, which began on April 4, 2004, will test the vaccine in approximately 450 healthy adults between the ages of 18 and 64. This trial is already fully enrolled and the safety data are being analyzed. If data from this study indicate the vaccine is safe and able to stimulate a certain immune response, NIAID expects to test the vaccine in other populations, such as the elderly and children, in late summer 2005. Trials of the Chiron-produced vaccines are expected to begin later this year.

In addition to these relatively small pilot lots, DHHS contracted with Sanofi-Pasteur to produce two million doses of its H5N1 vaccine, in order to ensure that the manufacturing techniques, procedures, and conditions that would be used for large-scale production will yield a satisfactory product. Moving to large-scale production of the vaccine in parallel with clinical testing of pilot lots is an indication of the urgency with which we have determined that H5N1 vaccine development must be addressed. Waiting for the results of the initial clinical trials, which would be the normal procedure, would delay our ability to make large quantities of vaccine by at least six months. These doses, which have now been delivered, could be used to vaccinate health workers, researchers, and, if indicated, the public in affected areas.

From the mid 1970s to the early 1990s, researchers in the NIAID Laboratory of Infectious Diseases developed a cold-adapted, live attenuated influenza vaccine strain that later became the FDA-licensed influenza vaccine marketed as FluMist. Building on their experience with attenuated influenza vaccines, researchers from the same laboratory recently made three candidate attenuated H5N1 vaccine strains and an attenuated H9N2 vaccine strain that are now in advanced development. NIAID plans to start the clinical trial of the attenuated H9N2 candidate vaccine this summer. These researchers also hope to test one of the candidate attenuated H5N1 vaccines in a Phase I study this year.

Antiviral Therapies

Antiviral medications are an important counterpart to vaccines as a means of controlling influenza outbreaks, both to prevent illness after exposure and to treat infection after it occurs. Four drugs are currently available for the treatment of influenza, three of which are also licensed for prevention of illness. NIAID actively supports identification of new anti-influenza drugs through the screening of new drug candidates in cell culture systems and in animal models. In the past year, seven promising candidates have been identified. Efforts to design drugs that precisely target viral proteins and inhibit their functions also are under way. In addition, NIAID is developing novel, broad-spectrum therapeutics that might work against many influenza virus strains. Some of these target viral entry into human cells, while others specifically attack and degrade the viral genome.

Efforts also are underway to test and improve antiviral drugs to prevent or treat H5N1 influenza. Last year, researchers determined that although H5N1 viruses are resistant to two older drugs—rimantadine and amantadine—they are sensitive to a newer class of drugs called neuraminidase inhibitors, including oseltamivir, which is marketed as Tamiflu. DHHS has stockpiled approximately 2.3 million treatment courses of oseltamivir, which is approved for use in individuals older than one year. Scientists are planning to conduct studies to further characterize the safety profile of oseltamivir in infants; and studies are also in progress to evaluate novel drug targets, as well as long-acting next-generation neuraminidase inhibitors. In addition, development and testing in animals of a combination antiviral regimen against H5N1 and other potential pandemic influenza strains are under way.

CONCLUSION

In closing, Mr. Chairman, I would like to emphasize that although we cannot be certain exactly when the next influenza pandemic will occur, we can be virtually certain that one will occur and that the resulting morbidity, mortality, and economic disruption will present extraordinary challenges to public health authorities around the world. We are working diligently in close coordination with our colleagues at CDC, FDA, other federal agencies, and in industry to ensure that we can meet these challenges in the most successful manner possible.

Thank you for this opportunity to appear before you today, and I would be pleased to answer any questions you may have.

Mr. DEAL. Thank you, Doctor. Dr. Gellin.

Mr. GELLIN. Thank you. I want to join my colleagues in thanking you for having this hearing.

Mr. DEAL. Can you pull that one a little closer?

STATEMENT OF BRUCE G. GELLIN

Mr. GELLIN. I want to thank you for holding this hearing because it is something that you and we and all the Americans really need to know about, as Ms. Baldwin mentioned. I am the Director of the National Vaccine Program Office, which sits in the Office of the Secretary of the Department of Health and Human Services. And I want to join my colleagues here to thank you for this.

As we have heard and you have been aware, the ecology of the disease and the behavior of the virus changing now offers multiple opportunities that could provide fertile ground for a pandemic virus to emerge. And while we are all keeping a watchful eye on the current situation in Asia, we recognize that there are other strains of the influenza virus that could perform similar tricks. And therefore, in addition to our focus on this virus, we acknowledge that a pandemic could be triggered by another influenza virus subtype and could originate in any country.

Secretary Leavitt has made pandemic influenza preparedness a priority area, and it is a critical component of his 500-day plan for the department. As Dr. Gerberding mentioned, just last week at the World Health Assembly in Geneva, the annual meeting of the ministers of health from around the world, he emphasized his concern about the situation in Asia and our department's and our government's commitment to preparedness. He encouraged global transparency, expanded surveillance, and timely sharing of information and clinical specimens, the importance that all nations have pandemic preparedness plans. He also urged international collaboration among developed and developing countries to control the spread of this virus and recognize the important role of the human-animal interface.

On the home front last summer, as we have heard and will discuss later, we released our draft plan last summer. The plan described a coordinated strategy to prepare for and respond to an influenza pandemic. It also provides guidance to State and local health departments and the healthcare system to enhance planning and preparedness at levels where the primary response activities in the U.S. will be implemented.

When we posted our plan, we sought public input before developing final guidance, and therefore allow the 60-day comment period for that. In addition, the National Vaccine Advisory Committee and CDC's Advisory Committee on Immunization Practices are currently discussing with a number of stakeholders to provide the department with recommendations on some key policy issues that are outstanding.

As a complement to the plant, CDC is also finalizing a series of specific guidance documents for State and local health departments, communities, and the healthcare system. We expect the updated plan and the related implementation guidance documents will be available in the coming months, but also recognize that plans like these will continue to evolve as we learn more. Therefore, we expect that we will regularly and continually review and revise the plan that incorporates new research, changing influenza strains, the changing epidemiology, lessons learned from the influenza season, and other infections disease threats.

In addition, we also recognize the importance that all Americans become aware of the threat of a pandemic and have begun to engage a number of public engagement and education projects because we seek the public's input into some of these decisions that we are making as well.

Moving ahead with our preparedness isn't waiting for the final drafting of the plan, as we have heard from both Dr. Fauci and Dr. Gerberding. And given the central role that vaccines play in preventing influenza, one of the critical elements of our plan is to develop a strategy for sufficient domestic surge capacity for vaccine production.

Our planning assumptions acknowledge that in a pandemic emergency, there is likely to be worldwide demand for vaccine, and vaccine produced outside the United States might not be available for our use. One of the base assumptions that we have in our planning is that the population has never be exposed to a virus or anything like this, and therefore, all may be susceptible, and therefore, all may need to be vaccinated.

And perhaps most importantly from a preparedness perspective, because it is the nature of the virus to evolve and re-assort with other influenza viruses, the perfect vaccine cannot be prepared far in advance and stockpiled since that vaccine is one that needs to be tailored to match the circulating strain.

As Dr. Fauci has mentioned with his discussion of the NIH clinical trials, HHS has developed a number of influenza vaccine supply initiatives to address pandemic preparedness needs, but will also be critical to achieving our annual influenza prevention goal. The objectives of these initiatives are to secure and expand U.S. influenza vaccine supply, diversify our production methodology, and establish emergency surge capacity. To support these activities HHS received $50 million in fiscal year 2004 and $99 million in fiscal year 2005. The 2006 budget includes an additional $120 million to further strengthen this component of our overall pandemic preparedness efforts.

To assure that vaccines can be produced at full manufacturing capacity at any time of the year, we also need to assure that we had an egg supply that could be available at any time of the year. And last year HHS issued a contract with sanofi pasteur that assures that they can manufacture influenza vaccine at their full capacity all year long.

But diversifying influenza vaccine production methods will also strengthen our system. As Dr. Fauci has mentioned, the cell-culture technology is a well-established vaccine production method for other vaccines and one that we hope can be applied effectively to influenza vaccine production. This technology does not require eggs as a substrate for growth and therefore avoids some of the vulnerabilities that are associated with that. And it also may be more amenable to surge production for emergency vaccine production.

Because of this the secretary announced last month that the Department of Health had issued a 5-year contract with sanofi pasteur for $97.1 million to develop a cell culture vaccine. The goal is to accelerate the efforts to bring such a vaccine to the United States, that have the vaccine licensed by the FDA, and to have it produced within the borders of the United States.

These important steps to strengthen our influenza vaccine supply, for assuring the egg supply, and diversifying our expanding production capacity are to be followed this year by additional measures to increase influenza vaccine capacity and expand the number of vaccine doses and the number of manufacturers that could supply vaccine to the United States.

Supported by the influenza vaccine initiative in the fiscal year 2006 budget in our request for $120 million, our goals are to build on our cell culture efforts and encourage additional manufacturers to accelerate the development of cell culture vaccines, to develop new vaccines such as recombinant vaccines, to improve the efficiency of the existing manufacturing processes, which could increase the overall yield of vaccines and the amount produced, and to support research and development of strategies that will stretch the number of doses produced by decreasing the amount of virus antigen in each dose, therefore making more vaccine from the same amount of antigen.

Finally, I need to mention that coupled with the effort that Dr. Fauci mentioned, last year we went ahead and had two million doses of H5N1 vaccine produced, and we did in a time in the fall that wouldn't interfere with seasonal production. We wanted to make sure that a company was familiar with making such a vaccine in full-scale facilities, and it was the first project like this in the world. We are awaiting the results of the clinical trials to know best how to use and formulate such a vaccine.

We also recognize the important role of antiviral drugs in stemming a pandemic. We have ordered and have already received delivery of over two million doses of Tamiflu, and we are currently in discussions with the manufacturer, Roche, who you will hear from later today, to increase our national reserve of this antiviral drug.

Stemming the spread of an epidemic will require close coordination between agriculture and health sectors and among effected countries, donor nations, and international organizations. To that end we have a planning effort underway to develop a plan for the $25 million that was included in the fiscal year 2005 emergency supplemental to the Department of State with the HHS focusing on health projects, and USAID, our partner, focusing on projects on animal health.

Last week Dr. Gerberding and I were part of the U.S. delegation accompanying Secretary Leavitt to the World Health Assembly. Of the many discussions there, the one that best captures the concern and common purpose that we all have is summarized in Mr. Leavitt's remarks to his fellow ministers of health: "There is a time in the life of every problem when it is big enough to see and small enough to solve. For pandemic influenza preparedness, that time is now." Thank you.

[The prepared statement of Bruce G. Gellin follows:]

PREPARED STATEMENT OF BRUCE G. GELLIN, DIRECTOR, NATIONAL VACCINE PROGRAM OFFICE, OFFICE OF PUBLIC HEALTH AND SCIENCE, OFFICE OF THE ASSISTANT SECRETARY FOR HEALTH, U.S. DEPARTMENT OF HEALTH AND HUMAN SERVICES

Mr. Chairman and Members of the Subcommittee, I am pleased to appear before you today to discuss pandemic influenza and the measures the Department of Health and Human Service is taking to prepare for the next pandemic. As you may have heard from reports from last week's World Health Assembly, many public health experts believe the threat of a pandemic is now greater than it has been in decades. A report issued by the World Health Organization warns that the virus may be evolving in ways that increasingly favor the start of a pandemic. In addition the ecology of the disease and behavior of the virus have changed and are creating multiple opportunities for a pandemic virus to emerge. This is in large part because of the bird flu that is established and now endemic in many different species of birds across Asia. As these bird viruses continue to evolve and spread in animals, the possibility increases that an avian virus will mix with a human virus to cause a novel and easily transmitted influenza strain in humans. Since 1997, the avian flu has continued to evolve and has become increasingly lethal for an expanding number of species, including mammals, not just birds. Over the past year and a half, there have been 97 confirmed human cases of influenza in Asia (Vietnam, Thailand and Cambodia) cause by the H5N1 virus and over half of these people have died from their infection.

Secretary Leavitt has made pandemic influenza a priority area. Just last week, at the World Health Assembly—the annual meeting of Ministers of Health from around the world—he emphasized his concern about the situation in Asia and the Department's commitment to preparedness. He encouraged global transparency, expanded surveillance, and timely sharing of information and clinical specimens as part of our global preparedness. Secretary Leavitt also urged international collaboration among developed and developing countries to control the spread of this virus among humans and animals. Further, the Assembly considered a resolution on pandemic preparedness that was offered by the U.S. as a blueprint for action.

In addition, on the national front, the Department has been actively developing and formulating a Pandemic Influenza Preparedness and Response Plan. This Plan describes a coordinated strategy to prepare for and respond to an influenza pandemic. It also provides guidance to state and local health departments and the health care system to enhance planning and preparedness at the levels where the primary response activities in the U.S. will be implemented.

This Plan was released for public comment last summer and, as with all preparedness planning, the specifics of this plan will continue to evolve. HHS will continually be revising and reworking the plan to respond to events such as new research, changing influenza virus strains, and discussions with the many stakeholders—state and local health departments, the health care system, industry and the public.

Given the central role that vaccines play in preventing influenza, one of the critical elements of this Plan is to develop a strategy for sufficient domestic surge capacity for influenza vaccine production. This will require an ongoing and sustained commitment by HHS.

Because a pandemic is by definition the introduction and spread of an influenza virus to which humans have not previously been exposed, this has major implications for vaccine development and supply. In the setting of a pandemic, it is assumed that the pandemic virus will be a novel strain. First, the majority of the population is likely to be susceptible; immunologic naivety with the pandemic strain is likely to result in the need for a two-dose regimen for effective immunity. Unlike seasonal influenza epidemics, a pandemic could come at any time during the year, and may last longer than a single season such that booster dose(s) may be required to sustain immunity. Perhaps most importantly from a preparedness perspective, the perfect vaccine cannot be prepared far in advance and stockpiled, since the ideal vaccine is one that should be tailored to match the circulating virus

Further, as highlighted by the SARS experience, modern transportation and trade are likely to rapidly accelerate the global spread of influenza. As a consequence, our planning assumptions acknowledge that in a pandemic emergency, there will be worldwide demand for vaccine and vaccine produced outside of the United States may not be available for our use.

We are all keeping a watchful eye on the current situation in Asia while at the same time recognizing that, in recent years, there have also been outbreaks of avian influenza infections in Europe and in Canada associated with human infections cases caused by other influenza subtypes. Therefore, in addition to our concerns about the H5N1 virus in Asia, we acknowledge that a pandemic could be caused by another influenza virus subtype could originate in any country.

Though scientists in 1918 had very little idea of what was happening until it was too late, we have time—and still have time—to prepare for the next global pandemic, and we should consider ourselves warned. As Secretary Leavitt stated at the World Health Assembly, "We are working on pandemic preparedness on borrowed time. When this event occurs, our response has got to be immediate, comprehensive and effective."

I want to assure you that the Department has made this one of its highest priorities and it is a critical component of the Secretary's 500-day plan. Ensuring the ability to meet current annual demand for influenza vaccine, to improve the prevention of influenza disease, and to prepare for an influenza pandemic all require strengthening the influenza vaccine supply in the U.S. Building on the response to the influenza vaccine shortage in the 2004-05 season NIH and FDA have worked to facilitate the clinical evaluation in U.S. populations of an influenza vaccine produced by GSK, and efforts are underway to expeditiously consider a licensure application such that this influenza vaccine may be licensed in the U.S. for the upcoming season.

Several HHS influenza vaccine supply initiatives have a longer timeline and were developed to address pandemic preparedness needs but which also will be critical to achieving annual influenza prevention goals. The objectives of these initiatives are to secure and expand U.S. influenza vaccine supply, diversify production methods, and establish emergency surge capacity. To support these activities, HHS received $50 million in FY2004 and $99 million in FY2005. The President's Budget for FY2006 includes an additional $120 million to further strengthen this component of the overall pandemic influenza preparedness efforts.

Because influenza vaccine is produced to meet the seasonal demand in the fall, production also is seasonal and embryonated eggs have not been available to manufacturers year-round. Moreover, although some excess supply of eggs may be available to support additional influenza vaccine production or provide security if the flocks that produce eggs for vaccine production are affected by avian influenza or other illness, this excess is limited creating vulnerability to supply disruption. To enhance influenza vaccine supply security, HHS issued a five-year contract to Sanofi-Pasteur of Swiftwater, Pennsylvania, on September 30, 2004 for $40.1 million. Under this contract, Sanofi-Pasteur has begun to change its flock management strategy to provide a secure, year-round supply of eggs suitable for influenza vaccine production at full manufacturing capacity. It also will increase the number of egg-laying flocks by 25% to provide contingency flocks in case of an emergency. These eggs may be used to support additional production of annual influenza vaccine in the event of a vaccine shortage. Additionally, this contract provides for production of annual investigational lots of prototype pandemic influenza vaccines, e.g., this summer, Sanofi-Pasteur will manufacture an H7N7 virus vaccine for clinical evaluation.

Diversification of influenza vaccine production methods also will help strengthen the system. Cell culture technology is a well-established vaccine production method for other vaccines such as the inactivated poliovirus vaccine and two companies have registered their cell-culture based influenza vaccine technology in Europe. This production technology does not require eggs as a substrate for growth of vaccine virus, thereby avoiding the vulnerabilities associated with an egg-based production system. It also may be more amenable to surge capacity production when influenza vaccine supply needs to be expanded rapidly such as at the time of a pandemic. Finally, influenza vaccines produced in cell cultures rather than eggs will provide an option for people who are allergic to eggs and therefore unable to receive the currently licensed vaccines.

Secretary Leavitt announced last month that the Department of Health and Human Services issued a five-year contract on March 31, 2005 to Sanofi-Pasteur for $97.1 million to develop cell culture influenza vaccine technology and conduct clinical trials, with the goal of obtaining an FDA license for this vaccine. Under this advanced development contract, the company has also committed to manufacturing this vaccine at a U.S.-based facility with a capacity to manufacture 300 million doses of monovalent pandemic vaccine over a one-year period. However, given timelines for vaccine development and clinical trials, and for construction and validation of manufacturing facilities, additional influenza vaccine supply from this source is unlikely to be available for at least five years.

These important steps to strengthen our national influenza vaccine supply through assuring the egg-supply and diversifying and expanding production capacity will be followed this year by additional measures to increase influenza vaccine production capacity and expand the number of influenza vaccine doses made using that capacity. Supported by the pandemic influenza vaccine initiative in the FY 2006 budget request for $120 M, we posted synopses of three additional areas where we believe strategic investments move us toward achieving annual and pandemic influenza vaccine supply goals in the March 17, 2005 edition of FedBizOpps. On April 29, 2005, the first of these requests for proposals was posted, providing support for the development of cell-culture based and recombinant pandemic influenza vaccines.

Whereas building new influenza vaccine production facilities is one approach to expand the influenza vaccine supply, other strategies also can increase the number of influenza vaccine doses produced. Influenza vaccine is manufactured in a series of steps—developing an influenza virus master seed for vaccine production, inoculating the virus into eggs, growing, harvesting, purifying, splitting, formulating, and filling it into vials or syringes. Improving efficiency at any step in this process can increase the eventual yield and number of vaccine doses produced. Thus, a second area of emphasis will be to support improvements of the manufacturing process to increase overall influenza vaccine production at current manufacturing facilities.

The third area of emphasis will provide support for research and development, leading to licensure of strategies that will stretch the number of vaccine doses produced by decreasing the amount of influenza virus antigen that is needed in each dose. The concept underlying these "dose-stretching" strategies is that by changing either the influenza vaccine or the way its administered, one can improve the immune response to vaccination and provide protection while using less of the vaccine antigen. By using less antigen in each vaccine dose, the number of doses that can be made at any level of production capacity can be multiplied. The two most promising antigen-sparing approaches are either to add an adjuvant—a substance that stimulates the immune response to a vaccine formulation, or administering the vaccine into the skin (similar to the approach used in a skin test for Tb) where large numbers of potent immune cells are located. Both strategies have been evaluated in several clinical trials and have the potential to expand influenza vaccine supply several-fold if they prove effective in further clinical trials and are approved for licensure.

The increases in the FY 2006 President's Budget request will support ongoing activities to ensure that the Nation will have an adequate influenza vaccine supply to respond better to yearly epidemics and to influenza pandemics. While issuing the requests for proposals and completing the contracts is only the first step toward the development of an expanded, diversified, and strengthened influenza vaccine supply, the U.S. is leading the global effort to develop vaccines and vaccine technologies to meet this challenge.

We also recognize the important role of antiviral drugs in stemming a pandemic and for treating patients. The United States has ordered and received delivery of 2.3 million treatment courses of Tamiflu. We are in discussions with Roche, the maker of Tamiflu ®, to increase our national reserve of this antiviral. Unfortunately, the H5N1 virus is resistant to the adamantine drugs, the only other class of anti-influenza drugs.

Stemming the spread of the epidemic will require close coordination between the agriculture and health sectors and among affected countries, donor nations and international organizations dedicated to promoting the health of humans, livestock and wildlife. Detailed joint planning is already underway to develop the proposed budget plan for the $25 million that was included in the FY 2005 emergency supplemental with the Department of State with HHS focusing on human health projects and USAID focusing on projects on animal health and related issues. In this way, the two agencies' plans will be complementary, not duplicative.

I was part of the U.S. delegation that attended last week's World Health Assembly and want you to know that this administration and the global health community are working together on this public health threat in anticipation of the next pandemic, be it tomorrow or ten years from now. As Secretary Leavitt told the assembled in Geneva, "There is a time in the life of every problem when it is big enough to see and small enough to solve. For pandemic influenza preparedness, that time is now."

Thank you for your attention to my remarks this morning—and more importantly to the attention that you are paying to this important global public health issue.

I would be happy to answer any questions from the Committee.

Mr. DEAL. Thank you. I recognize myself for some opening questions. It appears that we are now sort of focusing on the H5N1 as the flu that we think might be the one most likely to occur in pandemic form. Suppose we are wrong and it is the H9. Will vaccines that are developed for the H5 be effective for H9? Let me go ahead and ask a few series of questions and then I will let whoever wants to respond. That is the first question I have.

Second, are there antivirals that are being developed for this H5N1 or are antivirals somewhat generic in nature? Can they be used for any variation of strains or must they likewise be specific to the strain that we are facing?

The last two questions are is HHS contemplating stockpiling injection devices that would be needed in the event of a pandemic?

And last, I understand that there were some conditions in trying to trace the SARS issue that CDC faced in terms of being able to obtain passenger contact information. Have we overcome those administrative difficulties so that HHS or any other Federal agency would be able to provide the information necessary to trace someone who potentially has the H5 or any other variation of that virus coming into our country? I know that is a lot of questions and I will let you start.

Mr. GELLIN. Well, actually, you have a question for each of us.

Mr. DEAL. Okay.

Mr. GELLIN. Let me attack the vaccine and antiviral development one. You ask a very good question. The short answer to the question if you have an H5N1 vaccine, and, for example, an H9N2 virus circulating, the degree of protection would be minimal if none at all. So that is a clear answer to that question. I would point out in relationship to that question that for that very reason we are not just doing the trial with an H5N1. We have already started an H9N2 trial in much the same philosophy of looking at safety and proper doses of the H9N2.

Having said all that, if it is something else that is not H9N2 or not H5N1, the very fact of getting more experience with how the body responds to an antigen like an H5 or an H9 to which there have not been previous exposure will give us a lot of important information to more rapidly respond to whatever evolving Bird Flu, whatever the subtype is. So that is the answer to the question, but it also—the two million doses of the H5N1 allowed us to be able to make this kind of a vaccine in scale-up quality. So even though we are doing things now that might not be precisely matched to the ultimate pandemic flu virus, everything we are doing is going to helpful for that.

With regard to the antivirals, Tamiflu is the antiviral to which H5N1 is sensitive. The issue of developing antiviruses that have a broad range of capability is part of the research plan, as is developing vaccines that have broader capability, not to be only effective against one but against another. That is something that is difficult scientifically to do, but it is very high on our research agenda to do that.

And finally, with regard to the antiviral ability to block the influenza, we have to be very careful that there is not a perception that this is like an antibiotic that you treat pneumonia. You give it and the pneumonia is gone. This will maybe decrease some of the days of illness and be very, very useful, but we don't want you to get the impression that this is a knockout drop for the virus. It is not. And we have other questions that Dr. Gerberding will be able——

Ms. GERBERDING. The question about syringes is one that is easy to answer. We have a supply of a lot of medical equipment in the stockpile, and we are not concerned about shortages of syringes limiting immunization. The exact contents of the entire medical stockpile is something that we consider sensitive, so we would be happy to discuss with you in chambers the very specific contents of the stockpile.

And with respect to the issues around contacting passengers, our Division of Global Migration and Quarantine has been working with leaders at HHS and the administration to come up with some policies and procedures that would improve that process. Right now we are engaged in a pilot project with one major international airline to see if the data systems protect the confidentiality of the passengers but do allow this kind of reconnection. And we have already had one, I think, small event where it has been tested. It looks very promising. So we are taking an evidence-based approach to this. Find out a) does it work, b) is it acceptable to passengers, and c) can we do it at a cost that makes it a worthwhile investment. And we will know more about that probably later this year.

Mr. DEAL. Thank you. Mr. Brown.

Mr. BROWN. Thank you, Mr. Chairman. Dr. Gerberding, GO testified that insufficient hospital and health workforce capacity is a substantial area of concern. If you would, share with us your characterization of the adequacy of our hospital and health workforce capacity to deal with a potential pandemic, and if you think there are gaps, would you point us to specific provisions in the fiscal 2006 budget that are aimed at addressing these gaps?

Ms. GERBERDING. I will do my best to address that, and I may have to call upon Dr. Gellin to add perspective from the other agency that is involved in that, which is HRSA. I think we appreciate that our entire healthcare system lacks surge capacity for any kind of a major health issue. Workforce retention, development, recruitment, and training are issues that we all have a generic concern about. Since the terrorism preparedness investments have been

made by HHS, we have been able to target some specific preparedness activities to support surge capacity, and this year proposed in
the stockpile funding is money for portable hospital facilities of a
variety of levels of care so that we could bring portable facilities
to a site of a major event. And I will ask Mr. Gellin to add any
information from the HRSA perspective.

Mr. GELLIN. I think I will defer that and provide you that information in writing from HRSA so we are precise about it.

Mr. BROWN. Okay. Could you fill us in on your discussions with
the administration and their responses when you talk about the
gaps or the inadequacies of public health structure's ability to deal
with a pandemic outbreak?

Ms. GERBERDING. I can summarize all of this by saying I think
Secretary Leavitt represents the administrative position very well
and the high priority he has put on this, as well as the investments
that are proposed in the President's 2006 budget to increase the
Vaccines for Children Program, increase the purchase of vaccines
in the 317 Program to allow CDC to buy a backfill—sort of an in-
surance policy by buying bulk monovalent and vaccine in worst-
case scenario, to increase the ability of the States to purchase vaccine, as well as to change the Vaccines for Children Program to increase access for underinsured children to receive vaccines. So all
of these are plus ups in the budget.

I just mention that this year CDC's influenza budget is $197 mil-
lion, and that is about a log larger than it was just a few years
ago. So we are seeing proposed investments that I think augment
and buildupon the investments that we are making for terrorism
preparedness in the States. The capacities, as you know, are part
and parcel of the same—detection, surveillance, investigation, communication, informatics, and alerting. So it is my experience that
the entire department, as well as the rest of the administration, is
engaged in influenza and working very hard to come up with a co-
gent approach that would serve as well and to do it as fast as we
can.

Mr. BROWN. You argue or suggest that support from our government is adequate—from Congress, appropriations are adequate,
perhaps, for what you do specifically at CDC on that level. What
do you see when you look at hospitals and hospital infrastructure
and its abilities? Do you see funding gaps there and funding problems there? Or do you see an adequate amount of resources that
they are getting from State and local and Federal Governments?

Ms. GERBERDING. I am concerned, but I don't have data to answer your question. Again, this is a part of HRSA responsibility
that we can provide you a factual representation of the degree of
support and where the gaps might lie.

Mr. BROWN. Do the other two of you want to comment on that
or just simply something written? Okay. Thank you, Mr. Chairman.

Mr. DEAL. Thank you. Mr. Ferguson.

Mr. FERGUSON. Thank you, Mr. Chairman. Dr. Gerberding, I am
interested that in your statement or just your comments this morning that you didn't talk about antivirals really. You were talking
about vaccines. But can you talk a little about the role that

antivirals will play in an Avian Flu outbreak and in any kind of a pandemic flu outbreak?

Ms. GERBERDING. I think it is important to distinguish the H5N1 situation that we are looking at right now in Asia with the realm of possible influenza outbreaks that may occur. This particular virus strain happens to be resistant to the inexpensive, easily produced drugs. So if our only goal was to protect against this specific strain, stockpiling the other drugs doesn't make sense. But there are many other strains of flu that are susceptible to the inexpensive drugs. So we have made the decision to stockpile both categories of drugs. We are emphasizing oseltamivir right now because it is the drug most likely to be useful if this particular strain breaks. But we also have a stockpile of about four million treatment courses of rimantadine, which could be used for seasonal flu of a susceptible nature, or even an Avian strain that proved to be susceptible.

The problem with this antiviral stockpiling and capability can be summarized in the phrase "lack of evidence." We know that antiviral drugs, as Dr. Fauci said, can reduce the severity of illness as characterized by days of hospitalization and can benefit people if they are taken within 2 days of the onset of illness, which is very, very hard to do. You know, when you start getting the flu it is hard to distinguish it from any other upper respiratory infection, so most people don't realize they have flu until it is past the 48-hour window.

But in addition, we do not have evidence that even oseltamivir actually reduces mortality from influenza. The studies simply haven't been done. We are concerned at some of the things we are seeing in Vietnam where some patients who apparently were started early on the drug have not done well and have gone on to die despite treatment. So we need the scientific evidence to tell us how should the drug be used? Does it actually reduce mortality? What is its role in a pandemic? We are working with WHO and others in the department, including the FDA. We have been having regular conversations on how we might be able to conduct such trials in a situation where cases right now are still sporadic.

But until we actually know how to use the drugs, making enormous purchases in stockpiling may be a premature decision. And that is why we are scaling up our purchase as we feel we can define an effective role, but we have more work to do to really look at all the information and make the best possible long-term decision.

One other point I should make is that this right now is an oral drug. It is taken by mouth. And some of the patients with severe influenza in Asia have an illness that is not just respiratory in nature. It involves the GI tract and all other organs, and so we have to be concerned could this drug even get absorbed from the intestinal tract if people are ill with influenza. So we have a lot of work to do to be able to define the appropriate role for saving lives during flu and that work needs to be a high priority.

Mr. FERGUSON. But clearly our government is placing some new importance on the role of antiviral. We are going to hear more about antivirals in our next——

Ms. GERBERDING. Absolutely.

Mr. FERGUSON. [continuing] panel.

Ms. GERBERDING. Absolutely.

Mr. FERGUSON. And we are beginning to order millions and millions of doses I am told by some of the companies. To me it highlights that there is an increased awareness and appreciation for the role that antivirals can play.

Ms. GERBERDING. Yes, we have a stockpile right now of more than two million treatment courses of the oseltamivir, and with the supplemental appropriation we just received through the defense funding, the $58 million will be looking at what we might do with that resource to augment our stockpile also.

Mr. FERGUSON. I am sure you would agree with me that two million doses is a pittance. I mean that is nothing compared to what we would need were we to have some sort of a pandemic flu outbreak. But let me just—because my time is running short. I mean I think last year's vaccine shortage highlighted the question of the distribution—partnership that is going to be necessary, and even if we are stockpiling vaccines, stockpiling antivirals, what kind of a plan is in place and who is ultimately responsible for making sure the plan works to make sure that—I mean it could be because you are talking—I think the necessity of a 2-day window for someone to take an antiviral if they are showing signs of a flu, that I think highlights to me the necessity of having a distribution plan in place where these products are available and around the country. They are not all kind of sitting in one storehouse somewhere in one city or one part of the country that that—I mean it highlights to me that we need to have a real distribution plan in place. Can you shed some light on that?

Ms. GERBERDING. Any doctor can prescribe oseltamivir today, and it is available. We inventoried during last flu season. It is available in most pharmacies and could be readily available up to the amount that the manufacturer produces. So right now the commercial distribution system does a very good job of covering the United States. If we have stockpile drug and we need to allocate it in a setting of a flu pandemic, we would have some time to do that. We wouldn't expect instantaneously everyone in the country to be ill at the same time. So we would be able to distribute drugs in collaboration with the State health departments and others who have that primary responsibility depending on where the need was the greatest.

But that is part of the reason why we would like to have a larger stockpile, because the more pre-deployment we have in the system, the easier it is to handle that when people are frightened and upset.

I should also say that we are evaluating a number of options to support or augment distribution, including options that have been explored for terrorism events where countermeasures have to be delivered very quickly. One of those mechanisms involves working with the U.S. Postal Service to deliver products to people's homes. Another option might even include the idea of having the drugs forward-deployed at the community level or even the household level. So these are all things that are on the table right now, and we are working with experts inside and outside of government to come up with some evidence and some protocols to see which really will be the best approach.

Mr. FERGUSON. Mr. Chairman, I know my time is up, but just for me to close, I think it is important that we not underestimate the importance of antivirals in this process. And some of your comments suggest that perhaps you don't have the same appreciation that I might have or some folks at the World Health Organization. Their recommendation has been that, you know, countries have the ability to treat 25 to 50 percent of their population with antivirals. If we are talking about two million—even if we were talking about 50 million doses, that would not be enough. That would not be meeting the World Health Organization's recommendation so——

Ms. GERBERDING. But let——

Mr. FERGUSON. [continuing] I would urge you to look closer at some of those recommendations and perhaps take them to heart.

Ms. GERBERDING. Let me just be very clear. We do support stockpiling antivirals; we do think they have a role. We have defined the role of antivirals right now as one for treating affected people, and in certain situations, as a preventative for mission-critical personnel. We know the drug is effective at preventing seasonal flu, but obviously no one can treat the entire world with oseltamivir during the many, many months of a pandemic. So prophylaxis for the population is not sensible.

But I also wanted to emphasize, even those who are making projections about the proportion of population that should be covered are not doing that from a data base perspective or for—in some cases even credible models of how the drug would be used and distributed. So we have a lot of work to do to create a frame and a plan that includes antivirals in the context of other measures that must play a role, including isolation of cases and quarantine of exposed people.

Mr. FERGUSON. Thank you, Mr. Chairman.

Mr. DEAL. Thank you. As you know from the bells, we have a vote that is going on on the floor, and I want to commend the audience; I don't think I have heard a cough yet. We will resume as soon as these votes are concluded, and there are a series of votes, so we will be gone—yes.

Ms. ESHOO. If I could just ask my question, and I think I am next because I have another hearing of——

Mr. DEAL. Can you do it quickly?

Ms. ESHOO. I can do it very quickly.

Mr. DEAL. Okay.

Ms. ESHOO. To Dr. Gerberding, the GAO requested a plan, as I understand it, in 2000. And what I heard you say in your opening statement is that even though there has been a temporary report that has been issues, that you are just going to move ahead without doing a final report? I mean, I think that there is a little bit of a—I sense a conflict between what we need, what has been requested, a temporary report, all the needs that have been stated today, and how these conflicts or the differences or the gaps between a temporary report and a final report to the Congress, I am concerned about that because it really comes under the umbrella of a plan for our country. So you can either respond now or respond in writing.

And, Dr. Fauci, your testimony today, again, represents a great deal of hope, very exciting research and I think that it is good news for our country and that we are moving ahead. So if you——

Ms. GERBERDING. I would like to answer——

Ms. ESHOO. [continuing] address yourself——

Ms. GERBERDING. [continuing] your question quickly——

Ms. ESHOO. [continuing] to this because I am concerned about the, you know, the stated commitment but the lack of a plan and a timeframe for it.

Ms. GERBERDING. I think it is very important to understand how preparedness works. A plan would not necessarily be a good idea because look at all of the things that have happened in the last——

Ms. ESHOO. Well, why——

Ms. GERBERDING. [continuing] year——

Ms. ESHOO. [continuing] wasn't that stated when the GAO requested one?

Ms. GERBERDING. Well, I am not sure what the GAO is thinking, but we are intent on having a framework so that we can continuously update and improve. And I will ask Dr. Gellin because this plan right now is in his hands. And we are very intent on getting the stakeholders who have to execute the plan——

Ms. ESHOO. So there is a——

Ms. GERBERDING. [continuing] to have a voice in that process.

Ms. ESHOO. [continuing] temporary plan now and you are moving toward a final plan? And is that——

Ms. GERBERDING. There are elements of the plan that we already all agree on, and we are acting on those elements. There——

Ms. ESHOO. Will there be——

Ms. GERBERDING. [continuing] are some elements——

Ms. ESHOO. [continuing] a final plan?

Ms. GERBERDING. [continuing] that still have to be worked out. One of them——

Ms. ESHOO. Will there be a final plan——

Ms. GERBERDING. [continuing] was mentioned——

Ms. ESHOO. —Dr. Gellin, which will then be brought back and reported to the Congress, and if so, when?

Mr. GELLIN. Well, there will be a final plan in the sense that these plans are evergreen and that we know that they will continue to be revised. That said, I think the distinction between the moving ahead versus the final plan is more of how we are addressing the pandemic threats. You have heard from Dr. Gerberding and Dr. Fauci many of the specifics going into things that we are doing now because we are so concerned about the threat of the H5N1 virus and the bubbling up of other viruses around the world.

But the plan itself, as I mentioned, was lacking a few key policy decisions, but we put it out for public comment and we were seeking the input from others because we felt this was so important and it could affect every American, we wanted everyone potentially engaged in that. So while a large part of that framework is completed, some of those components, the distribution and control of vaccines, as we were just talking about——

Ms. ESHOO. But do you have a plan for a final plan? When do you anticipate——

Mr. GELLIN. Plan for——

Ms. ESHOO. [continuing] bringing back——
Mr. GELLIN. This summer.
Ms. ESHOO. [continuing] something that is——
Mr. GELLIN. This summer.
Ms. ESHOO. [continuing] rounded out——
Mr. GELLIN. As I mentioned there are a number——
Ms. ESHOO. [continuing] but perhaps to this committee——
Mr. GELLIN. Sure.
Ms. ESHOO. [continuing] which has jurisdiction.
Mr. GELLIN. Well, we would be happy—we will post it for the world on our website and we will share with the World Health Organization when it is available. We would be glad to come and talk to you about it as well. We expect it will be completed——
Ms. ESHOO. Do you anticipate approximately——
Mr. GELLIN. This summer.
Ms. ESHOO. [continuing] when?
Mr. GELLIN. This summer.
Ms. ESHOO. I mean is it 2 years from now or a year——
Mr. GELLIN. This summer.
Ms. ESHOO. This summer?
Mr. GELLIN. This summer. As I said, there are a number of moving parts that are going to funnel into it, and we are hopeful that they are all going to be completed. The CDC is working on some, various advisory committees are working on them, and they are all anticipated to funnel in to fill the few gaps that were in the plan from last year this summer.
Ms. ESHOO. Thank you. Thank you, Mr. Chairman.
Mr. DEAL. Thank you. The committee stands in recess.
[Brief recess]
Mr. DEAL. The subcommittee will come back to order. I recognize Dr. Burgess for questions.
Mr. BURGESS. Thank you, Mr. Chairman. Dr. Gellin, on the issue of liability that inevitably comes up in a discussion like this, have you got any thoughts on the issue of liability and protection from liability that may enter into this discussion?
Mr. GELLIN. Well, specifically for this discussion, I think it is worth highlighting that the National Vaccine Injury Compensation Program that added the influenza vaccine to their compensation table this year added a trivalent vaccine, the current annual vaccine of three strains. And I believe that probably gives us some indication that a pandemic vaccine, which we all believe would likely be a monovalent strain of the pandemic strain wouldn't be covered by the compensation program. In my reading of the history of the Swine Flu epidemic in 1976, the manufacturers—I believe, and they will probably tell you about that—but produced vaccine but wouldn't release it until the liability question was solved. I think among the pieces of the preparedness plan, at least that have been highlighted as one that needs to be solved, is the one that is being worked on, but clearly needs to be solved before we can move forward. And a large response is that issue.
Mr. BURGESS. Thank you. And, Dr. Gellin, the vaccine shortage from last year, the utilization of information, lessons learned from that vaccine shortage, has that in any way helped us nationally plan for the pandemic flu response?

Mr. GELLIN. Absolutely. And I think that what your question really highlights is really the inseparable link between our annual influenza program and our preparedness for a pandemic. And that speaks probably to every component of that from communications to vaccine distribution to vaccine availability. So we learned many lessons last year. And I think that one of the other questions that needs to be addressed and is one of those key policy decisions that was intentionally left out of the plan because we wanted a larger discussion was the procurement and distribution and essentially the control of vaccine in a pandemic.

It is worth highlighting that while we all think about flu shots and public health and therefore you think that this must be a public commodity, 85 percent, I believe, of the flu shots that are distributed annually are in the private sector. And I think that what we saw some last year is that the control of vaccine was really an impairment to the distribution of vaccine. Therefore, I think we need a vigorous discussion that goes into our policy decisions about procurement and control of a pandemic vaccine.

Mr. BURGESS. Thank you. Dr. Gerberding, Dr. Fauci talked about fast science and how good we are now at identifying things. The concept of syndromic surveillances is something that comes up from time to time. Are we making any effort to tie into any of the large drugstore chains to see when the sales of Kleenex and aspirin spike so that we could even be a little bit faster about trying to identify these outbreaks?

Ms. GERBERDING. Thank you. During this past flu season we did test out our system called BioSense, which allows us to import information from pharmacies as well as clinical visits in the VA and the Department of Defense sites across the country, of course, anonymously without revealing patient identifiers and a number of other related, surrogate health data short of actual patient visits to the hospital or clinician for influenza. And what we found was that our inputted information from over-the-counter purchases of flu-type medications in conjunction with clinic visits in the Department of Defense and VA medical facilities allowed us in some jurisdictions to see the arrival of flu earlier than our conventional surveillance and with more precision at the local level than our conventional surveillance. For seasonal flu that is probably not particularly helpful to the public health and the doctors making the decisions, but in the case of something like exotic Avian Influenza or pandemic strain or SARS, the sooner we know that at the most local level, the sooner we can initiate isolation, quarantine, and other control measures. So we think this is definitely an investment that has proved its use, and we continue to evaluate it and improve it over the next year. So we actually appreciate the support that Congress has given us for the BioSense initiative.

Mr. BURGESS. Well, and also, of course, most of the agents that are discussed as far as Homeland Security, the bioterrorism agents would present with the same symptoms as an influenza outbreak?

Ms. GERBERDING. That is correct. There is always a dual purpose. Everything we do with flu helps us with terrorism preparedness and vice versa.

Mr. BURGESS. I guess, Dr. Gellin, Mr. Brown asked you about surge capacity in the provider market, and has there been any thought given to—you know, there are physicians out there who are licensed and capable but no longer insured because they might be retired, serving in Congress, any number of other occupations. And has there been any thought given to a limited liability protection during a crisis that would provide some of that surge capacity that you say we lack?

Mr. GELLIN. Well, I can't speak to that, but specifically for a pandemic response I don't know if that has been addressed in bioterrorism, but clearly we recognize that the kinds of numbers that you all have been aware of and have discussed with us, it would rapidly overwhelm the healthcare system and need to try to think of alternative levels of care and what it would take to allow that to happen.

Mr. BURGESS. Thank you. This has been a fascinating discussion this morning. I hope I can get continuing education hours. Thank you, Mr. Chairman.

Mr. DEAL. The gentleman from California, Mr. Waxman.

Mr. WAXMAN. My colleague wants not only continuing education but a legal liability protection if he is called into service. Not unreasonable. Not unreasonable at all. Dr. Gerberding, we are going to hear on the next panel from sanofi-aventis, the only company with a plant licensed to produce flu vaccine in the United States, and they also make several childhood vaccines, including vaccines to prevent polio, tetanus, and whooping cough. And the company is going to tell us that in the event of a pandemic, virtually all of their efforts would be directed toward a flu vaccine and production of other vaccines would plummet. Now, that might not be a problem if we have a stockpile of all the pediatric vaccines. Three years ago CDC pledged to fill this stockpile, but as the "Washington Post" recently reported, very little progress has been made. Over 2 years ago sanofi-aventis raised the concern with CDC that an obscure accounting rule of the Securities and Exchange Commission was an obstacle to participation. The SEC issue has since been discussed in advisory committee meetings and CDC presentations and scholarly publications, yet for all this talk, very little action. And I just learned that 2 days ago, the SEC sent its first letter to the vaccine companies asking for more information. The SEC is hoping the companies will call by June 7 in order to schedule a conference call or a meeting.

Now, if CDC was aware of the problem 2 years ago, why does it seem to be stuck at square one in May 2005, and what are you doing to express the urgency of this situation to Secretary Leavitt at HHS and Chairman Donaldson at SEC? When do you foresee this problem will be resolved? When can we expect the stockpile to be filled? This is not a complicated problem. We need vaccines for a stockpile so that we can protect children's lives. But the stockpile is now virtually empty and children are at risk, and if a high enough priority is placed on children's health by this administration, this problem should be able to be resolved I would think immediately. I know it is not your problem alone, but it is others' within the administration. When are we going to see action on this?

Ms. GERBERDING. This is a frustrating situation. For 20 years we have been purchasing drugs for the pediatric supply using a method that served us very well, and suddenly a couple of years ago, as you mentioned, the accounting rule was noticed or interpreted differently than it had in the past, and some companies are concerned enough to no longer want to stockpile drugs and vaccines using the old methodology.

We had a very difficult time getting an accountant with objectivity to help us because most of the accountants that we approached for contractual relationships have conflicts of interest because they also do work for PhRMA. So the process of getting the external advice and help that we needed took longer than you can imagine. It was a very frustrating situation, but the accountant is on board. We do have an objective accountant that I think we would all agree does not have a conflict of interest in how to arbitrate and negotiate a decision.

I will be frank with you; I am not an expert in Securities and Exchange law, but I know that Secretary Leavitt and the department have been working hard to try to find some alternative strategy. The reason that we have managed the stockpile in this way is because we don't want to purchase vaccine and have it expire and not use it——

Mr. WAXMAN. No, I understand that and——

Ms. GERBERDING. [continuing] so it is——

Mr. WAXMAN. [continuing] it must be——

Ms. GERBERDING. The solution is expensive——

Mr. WAXMAN. Yes.

Ms. GERBERDING. [continuing] and we are looking——

Mr. WAXMAN. Well, it must be——

Ms. GERBERDING. Isn't there some——

Mr. WAXMAN. [continuing] frustrating to you——

Ms. GERBERDING. [continuing] third way——

Mr. WAXMAN. [continuing] and it is frustrating to everybody involved. One person suggesting putting people in the room and not letting them out until they have resolved it. I want to express to you on my behalf, and maybe I speak for other members as well, if you need a special exemption in the law on this one issue in order to give comfort to the companies to produce the stockpile, if that is what it comes to, I would certainly support such an effort. So I just want to encourage you to push the secretary, who has so many other things on his mind, to not forget this one because it could blow up in our face.

The key Federal program that supports State immunization activities is the 317 Program. It supports basic childhood immunization as well as resources and training directly related to pandemic flu preparedness, and for years States have raised concerns about Federal support. They say 317 is inadequate. Spending for vaccine planning staff has remained flat even though costs have risen. More than 15 States say they don't have the resources to provide routinely recommended vaccines such as a vaccine against the most common cause of meningitis to all children who need it.

Last year Congress provided an extra $6 million for the 317 Program, but then that money had to be diverted when we had the flu crisis. States have said they are not seeing the increase in funding even though they were told they would get it. Is this extra funding going for vaccine purchase, and if not, where it is going?

I assume that is where it is going. Last fall CDC took money from the 317 Program to purchase flu vaccine. Has all the funding been restored to the 317 Program? Can you pledge that it will be fully restored?

Ms. GERBERDING. No, let me first say that use of 317 money for the IND vaccine has been fully restored, so we did not borrow from 317 on a permanent basis to pay for the vaccine. We reprogrammed through Congressional action to pay for those expenses through non-317 dollars. And overall there is a net increase in 317 support. I would also mention that we have record high immunization records of children across our Nation. So whatever difficulties the States are having, they have been able to get the best-ever vaccination rates in very difficult times, which I think is a testament to their incredible innovation and creativity under some pretty high pressure circumstances.

Mr. WAXMAN. So it is your position that there really has not been a decline in 317 funds? The money has been restored and it is available?

Ms. GERBERDING. There is an actual, absolute increase in the funding for 317. But the other part of this that hasn't been resolved yet is the change in the Vaccine for Children Program that would allow a population of children that right now experience a coverage gap. Uninsured children in the country cannot get vaccine through the 317 Program in the locations where we would like them to be able to access it. And we are supporting a change in vaccines for children that would cover those children under the mandatory vaccination program so they would no longer be relying on 317 funds. That should help improve coverage.

Mr. WAXMAN. Thanks. Well, it is an important program, and I just want to urge you to make sure that we have enough funds in there for the States to do their job.

Ms. GERBERDING. Thank you.

Mr. WAXMAN. Thank you. Thank you, Mr. Chairman.

Mr. FERGUSON [presiding]. As we are waiting for members of the majority side to come back we will go to Mr. Allen.

Mr. ALLEN. Thank you, Mr. Chairman. This is a question for the whole panel really. I am just wondering what your estimate is of the time it would take between identification of a pandemic strain and full-scale production of a vaccine against that strain? I know some assumption is built in there, but I wondered if you could give us your thoughts on that question.

Ms. GERBERDING. We face a similar situation every year because we see season flu emerge at the end of the regular flu season, and we have got to scale everything up to be able to produce the next vaccine for the fall. So 6 months is the best we can do right now under our current manufacturing processes. And part of the reason that the vaccine, the H5 vaccine, the two million doses is so important is because some of the regulatory steps to allow for good manufacturing practice approval, those hurdles have already been solved. And if we have to suddenly use the slightly different H5 strain or scale up the production of this one, we have cutoff a little bit of the regulatory barrier to the time. But egg production takes time. It takes time to get a seed virus and it takes time to grow it in eggs; it takes time to harvest it; it takes time to package it and test it and then distribute it. So we would have to count on a 6-month window before we would have full-scale global production.

Mr. FAUCI. Yes, I agree completely with Dr. Gerberding's estimate of the timeframe, Mr. Allen, but I would like to take the opportunity just for a few seconds to emphasize something I mentioned early on. And that is we should not assume that if we have a 6-month lead, if the virus evolves in a rather less-than-abrupt but more gradual way, which is likely that it would, and we press the button and say we are going to go full-scale now, even with that, the capacity for the number of doses we would have is still an important limiting factor. So it isn't as if overnight we are going to be able to get a vaccine for everyone who would need a vaccine. That is very important. The reason I bring it up—that is the bad news. The news that should spur us to do what we have spoken certainly to members of this committee before is by linking our preparedness for the regular, seasonal influenza with the preparedness for pandemic flu so that gradually we increase the usage of, the consistency of demand for, and the capacity for influenza vaccine such that we have a situation that on a regular year we are making 150 million, 180 million. That would put us in much better stead to be able to respond in a very quick way if we indeed have to respond to a pandemic flu. That is extremely important.

Mr. ALLEN. Okay. Thank you. Dr. Gellin, any difference of opinion?

Mr. GELLIN. No difference of opinion, but I want to sort of qualify and add a few things to what Drs. Gerberding and Fauci said. I think it is important to think about the entire timeframe. You signaled when it starts and when we have something. I think that really reinforces the importance of surveillance, to have the eyes, ears, and hands, and labs out there that can find that virus soon. And I think that we have gone ahead with this H5 projects, the several H5 projects really are evidence of that.

The other piece is recognizing that when vaccine starts to come off the line that it is going to take a while for it to come off, which is again why a system other than eggs where you can have multiple things going on in parallel so the time to the first dose may be the same, but the number of doses you get subsequently may be greatly increased.

Mr. ALLEN. Thank you. Let me do a related question. Because of concerns about how long it might take to develop a pandemic strain vaccine, the U.K. and France among other countries have already ordered sufficient supply of Tamiflu for about one-fourth of their population. And according to press reports, the U.S. has only ordered for 1 percent of the population. Should we create a larger stockpile of Tamiflu? What is the timetable for ordering more supply? And sort of what level of funding would be necessary to do that?

Ms. GERBERDING. We have made the decision to increase our stockpile. Again, part of the resources that came through the supplement just recently, the last couple of weeks, may be used to do that. And we also intend to purchase more stockpile materials to combat flu and——

Mr. ALLEN. Is there a number? About how much more do you think?

Ms. GERBERDING. I am not ready to give you an exact number today.

Mr. GELLIN. Let me make a distinction, which is important, because of what you have cited in the press. The difference between orders and actual what you have in stock, we have been worried about this for some period of time and went ahead and have secured the over two million treatment courses, enough to treat over two million people. And while other countries have signaled their intent to purchase more, it is going to be several years until that is delivered. I am sure the companies can fill you in on that. And in the meantime few are going to have to have a strategy to be able to prioritize those who would be first in line in a limited supply. But I think that is where our—we have actually emphasized both the antivirals and the vaccine, recognizing that these are the only two medical countermeasures that we might have, neither of them perfect, but we need to do what we could with both of them.

Mr. ALLEN. Thank you all.

Mr. FERGUSON. Ms. Baldwin.

Ms. BALDWIN. Thank you, Mr. Chairman. I wanted to further pursue two of the questions that I raised in my opening statement. First, regarding planning and preparedness on a global scale—and I was pleased to hear in your testimony about Secretary Leavitt addressing the World Health Assembly and elevating this issue.

Some of the experts at home and abroad have even gone as far as describing what a formalized global flu pandemic effort should look like, including some sort of global taskforce, outbreak management teams with some sort of centralized management. Is anything happening to achieve these right now, and does anything like what I have just described exist?

Ms. GERBERDING. Thank you. I attended the World Health Assembly with Dr. Gellin and Secretary Leavitt and others this year. I also attended the assembly last year, and I can tell you that there has been a sea change of interest and focus on influenza in the last year. The meetings were incredibly well-attended and some very specific actions, steps, and subsequent plans were laid out that I think will lead to action.

But what we are doing, in addition to what the World Health Organization is doing, is to use the supplemental resources that we were provided, $15 million this past week to CDC and another $10 million to USAID to specifically focus right now on Southeast Asia. And we are in the process of developing very specific capabilities that would include improving the local ability to identify cases and to get the frontline lab test done, as well as augmenting the training of the many health aids and clinicians and public health officials that would need to engage to improve the infrastructure, particularly in the Mekong Delta countries.

So we haven't finalized that plan; we are still working on it because we are working in collaboration with USAID and the Department of Defense as well as the Ministers of Health and the World Health Organization. But I think this is going to give us a giant step forward in our ability to do something right now in the region to really do exactly what you are suggesting needs to be done.

Mr. GELLIN. And if I could, I will just speak to that in a different way. The World Health Organization in 1999 put out the first Pandemic Influenza Preparedness Plan framework and asked that all countries follow that. As you can imagine, that would ease communication when people would have a similar understanding of where they were in a pandemic. They regionally revised that, and I think it was last December or January, which again forces us to change our plan, which speaks again to the fact that these plans will continue to evolve. But again the one that will come out this summer will follow the WHO framework.

I think it does speak to what Dr. Gerberding mentioned and reinforced that people recognize the definition of a pandemic is a global problem, and all the countries, those affected and those who might be affected, are in this together.

Ms. GERBERDING. I got the International Health Regulations approved at the World Health Assembly so member nations voted approval of new requirements that would mandate countries to report any condition that could pose an international health threat with specific mention of influenza and SARS-like illness.

Ms. BALDWIN. Thank you. The other issue that I wanted to pursue in greater depth—this question is for you, Dr. Gellin—is the component of public education preparedness in that sense. And I think back to how information was disseminated when we had the anthrax attacks, what level of preparation there was for that in terms of public awareness. And obviously there was certainly some elements of panic, et cetera. Tell me if you will—and you alluded to this in your testimony that there are elements in place and moving forward—what are they? What sort of strategies do you have to educate the public and maybe also working with the media?

Mr. GELLIN. Well, I think there is a lot that has begun to be put in place, and I guess I would actually put it in terms of a two-way discussion. Education sounds like we are going to tell you what we know, but we also want to have that as a discussion that goes both ways. So there are a number of things that are now being developed. There are going to be some—I mean I don't know if they are precisely town hall meetings, but ways to go out and have discussion with representatives of the public. I think part of the challenge is going to be the separation of pandemic influenza from regular influenza, recognizing the challenges of that every year.

And I think it was ironic that last year, when we put out our draft plan on August 26, it was the day that Chiron first announced that they were having trouble. So our intention to put that plan out away from the flu season specifically to try to separate pandemic influenza from influenza changed. But I think that we are probably all living with the fact that influenza and pandemic influenza seem to be everyday discussions.

Ms. BALDWIN. Have these town hall meetings begun to happen or are they in the pipeline? What——

Mr. GELLIN. In the pipeline. The——

Ms. GERBERDING. There are other things that have been going on as well. We have ongoing focus groups, particularly in follow-up to last year's flu vaccine. One critical question we need to know is will clinicians still want to offer flu vaccine. So we have been doing surveys to get answers to what will target audiences do under various circumstances of supply or severity of flu.

We have also, through out preparedness investments in the States, created a whole curriculum on risk communication, and all States now have risk communicators in the State Health Department or the Governor's office who are experienced at explaining things to the public in times of high stress and emotional conduct. And we have exercised those.

Unfortunately, many times in the last several months through the many non-flu-related outbreaks and tsunamis and hurricanes that we have experienced, but we are finding that capacity has grown dramatically since anthrax. We know from that kind of formative research that although government leaders are very important in setting the stage for the communication, the person that people most want to hear information from is their own doctor. And so targeting the clinicians as a component of the educational—it is absolutely critical at the local level.

Mr. FERGUSON. With that we will conclude our first panel. I want to thank our witnesses, Dr. Gerberding, Dr. Fauci, Dr. Gellin, thank you very much for being here today. Thank you for the work that you do on behalf of the healthcare of the American people. And I will invite the witnesses for our second panel to come to the witness table. I know Chairman Deal had introduced our second panel earlier in the hearing but very briefly by way of introduction, our second panel includes Dr. Marcia Crosse, the Director of Health Care Issues at GAO; Mr. Phillip Hosbach, Vice President of Immunization Policy and Government Relations at sanofi pasteur; Dr. Ralph Tripp, Professor and GRA Chair at the University of Georgia College of Veterinary Medicine, Department of Infectious Diseases; Dr. Andrew Pavia, Infectious Diseases Society of America; and Dr. Dominick Iacuzio, Medical Director at Hoffmann-La Roche. Thank you all very much for being here. We appreciate your presence. Dr. Crosse, we will begin with you. Just turn on your microphone if you would. Thank you.

STATEMENTS OF MARCIA CROSSE, DIRECTOR, HEALTH CARE ISSUES, UNITED STATES GOVERNMENT ACCOUNTABILITY OFFICE; ANDREW T. PAVIA, CHAIRMAN, TASKFORCE ON PANDEMIC INFLUENZA, INFECTIOUS DISEASES SOCIETY OF AMERICA, AND PROFESSOR AND CHIEF, DIVISION OF PEDIATRIC INFECTIOUS DISEASES, UNIVERSITY OF UTAH MEDICAL CENTER; PHILLIP HOSBACH, VICE PRESIDENT, IMMUNIZATION POLICY AND GOVERNMENT RELATIONS, SANOFI-PASTEUR; DOMINICK A. IACUZIO, MEDICAL DIRECTOR, HOFFMANN-LA ROCHE; AND RALPH A. TRIPP, CHAIRMAN, GEORGIA RESEARCH ALLIANCE, AND PROFESSOR, DEPARTMENT OF INFECTIOUS DISEASES, UNIVERSITY OF GEORGIA, COLLEGE OF VETERINARY MEDICINE

Ms. CROSSE. I am pleased to be here today as you discuss issues regarding our preparedness to respond to an influenza pandemic. We have heard today already about the threat posed by Avian Influenza. As many members noted, while the extent of the next pandemic cannot be predicted, modeling studies suggest that its effects in the United States could be severe.

You asked us to provide our perspective on the Nation's ability to conduct disease surveillance for an influenza pandemic, as well as preparedness for such a pandemic. In my testimony I will briefly discuss surveillance systems and the challenges that remain in preparedness and response.

There are a number of systems in place to identify influenza outbreaks abroad, to alert us to a pandemic, and these systems generally appear to be working well. HHS has taken important steps to enhance surveillance. Given the global nature of disease, a pandemic that begins abroad could quickly spread to this country. Public health officials plan to rely on the Nation's existing influenza surveillance system and recent enhancements to identify an influenza pandemic. CDC currently collaborates with multiple public health partners, as we heard, including WHO to obtain data that provide national and international pictures of influenza activity.

Public health officials and healthcare organizations have undertaken several initiatives that may be expected to enhance influenza surveillance. While some of these initiatives are focused more generally on increasing preparedness for bioterrorism and emerging infectious diseases, others have been undertaken specifically in preparation for an influenza pandemic. For example, in response to concerns over the past few years about Avian Influenza, CDC implemented an initiative in cooperation with WHO to improve influenza surveillance in Asia, which Dr. Gerberding discussed.

CDC has also implemented initiatives to improve public health communications systems it uses to collect and disseminate surveillance information for many diseases. In addition, CDC, FDA, and the Department of Agriculture have made efforts to enhance their coordination of surveillance efforts for animal diseases that can be transferred to humans such as SARS and certain strains of influenza.

While public health officials have undertaken several initiatives to enhance influenza surveillance capabilities, challenges remain with regard to other aspects of preparedness and response. The steps HHS is taking to address these challenges may not be in place in time to fill the current gaps in preparedness should an influenza pandemic occur in the next several years.

One area of concern is the supply of vaccine and antiviral drugs. As we learned in the 2004-2005 influenza season, the vaccine supply is fragile. It takes many months to produce vaccine and problems with even a single manufacturer can result in vaccine shortages.

Further, as was extensively discussed in the first panel, our current stockpile of antiviral drugs is insufficient to meet the likely demand in a pandemic. HHS is working to expand vaccine production capacity and to stockpile vaccine and antiviral drugs, but it will be years before these preparations are in place.

Other challenges in preparedness and response exist across the public and private sectors. Regulatory, privacy, and procedural issues surrounding measures to control the spread of disease must be addressed. And both the public and private sectors must resolve issues related to an insufficient hospital capacity and health workforce for responding to a large-scale outbreak such as an influenza pandemic. A pandemic would have major impacts on the ability of communities to respond, businesses to function, and public safety to be maintained.

Finally, since 2000 we have been urging the department to complete its pandemic plan. A draft plan was issued in August 2004, but the plan has not been finalized. Our concern is not whether the plan is modified and updated on the basis of experience or events, but absent a completed Federal plan, key questions remain unanswered. Some decisions yet to be made include: determining the Federal role and the public versus private sector role in the purchase, distribution, and administration of vaccines and antiviral drugs; how population groups will be prioritized for vaccination; what quarantine authorities or travel restrictions may need to be invoked; and how Federal resources should be deployed during a pandemic. It is important for the Federal Government and the States to work through these issues before we are in a time of crisis.

Mr. Chairman, this concludes my prepared statement. I would be happy to answer any questions you or other members of the subcommittee may have. Thank you.

[The prepared statement of Marcia Crosse follows:]

PREPARED STATEMENT OF MARIA CROSSE, DIRECTOR, HEALTH CARE, UITED STATES GOVERNMENT ACCOUNTABILITY OFFICE

Mr. Chairman and Members of the Subcommittee: I am pleased to be here today as you discuss issues regarding the nation's preparedness to respond to a worldwide influenza epidemic, or influenza pandemic.[1] The emergence of new diseases such as severe acute respiratory syndrome (SARS) has raised concerns about our ability to respond to other infectious disease outbreaks such as an influenza pandemic,[2] which many experts believe to be inevitable. Vaccine shortages and distribution problems during the 2004-2005 influenza season add to these concerns.

Influenza pandemics arise periodically but unpredictably from a major genetic change in the virus that results in a new strain.[3] Some experts believe that the next pandemic could be spawned by the recurring avian influenza in Asia. As of May 19, 2005, 97 people, mostly young and otherwise healthy, have been confirmed by the World Health Organization (WHO) to have been infected with avian influenza since 2003, and 53 of them have died. Recent studies suggest that avian influenza strains are increasingly capable of causing severe disease in humans and suggest that these strains have become endemic in some wild birds. If these avian influenza strains directly infect humans and acquire the ability to be readily transmitted between people, a pandemic could occur.

While the severity of the next pandemic cannot be predicted, modeling studies suggest that its effect in the United States could be severe. The Centers for Disease Control and Prevention (CDC) estimates that if a "medium-level" influenza pandemic were to occur in the United States, in the absence of any control measures (e.g., vaccination and drugs), it could cause 89,000 to 207,000 deaths, 314,000 to 734,000 hospitalizations, 18 million to 42 million outpatient visits, and another 20 million to 47 million cases of the illness.[4] From 15 percent to 35 percent of the U.S. population could be affected by an influenza pandemic, with associated costs ranging from $71 billion to $167 billion.

---

[1] An influenza pandemic is defined by the emergence of a novel influenza virus, to which much or all of the population is susceptible, that is readily transmitted person-to-person and causes outbreaks in multiple countries.

[2] See GAO, *SARS Outbreak: Improvements to Public Health Capacity Are Needed for Responding to Bioterrorism and Emerging Infectious Diseases,* GAO-03-769T (Washington, D.C.: May 7, 2003).

[3] Influenza pandemics can have successive "waves" of disease and last for up to 3 years. Three pandemics occurred in the 20th century: the "Spanish flu" of 1918, which killed 500,000 people in the United States; the "Asian flu" of 1957, which caused 70,000 deaths in the United States; and the "Hong Kong flu" of 1968, which caused 34,000 deaths in the United States.

[4] See CDC, *Fact Sheet, Information about Influenza Pandemics,* 3, www.cdc.gov/flu, downloaded May 12, 2005.

You asked us to provide our perspective on the nation's ability to conduct disease surveillance[5] for an influenza pandemic, as well as the public health system's preparedness for an influenza pandemic. In this testimony, I will discuss (1) surveillance systems in place to identify and monitor an influenza pandemic and (2) challenges in preparedness and response to an influenza pandemic.

My testimony today is based largely on our 2004 report on disease surveillance[6] as well as reports and testimony on influenza outbreaks, influenza vaccine supply, pandemic planning, and the SARS outbreak that we have issued since October 2000[7] and work we have conducted to update key information. Our prior work on disease surveillance and influenza pandemics included analysis of information provided by multiple federal departments and agencies, including the Department of Health and Human Services (HHS)—specifically from CDC and the Food and Drug Administration (FDA)—and the Departments of Agriculture, Defense, and Homeland Security, as well as interviews with officials of those departments and agencies. We also interviewed public health department officials from 11 states,[8] vaccine manufacturers, and vaccine distributors and surveyed physician group practices. To learn about pandemic planning efforts, we interviewed HHS officials in the National Vaccine Program Office and reviewed HHS's August 2004 draft "Pandemic Influenza Preparedness and Response Plan." Our prior work on the SARS outbreak included analysis of information provided by U.S. agencies, WHO, and Asian governments, as well as interviews with officials from those entities. We also conducted fieldwork on SARS in Beijing; Hong Kong; Guangdong Province, China; and Taipei, Taiwan. In May 2005, we updated our information to include issues that arose during the 2004-2005 influenza season and to verify the current status of HHS efforts on surveillance, planning, and preparedness activities. We conducted all of our work in accordance with generally accepted government auditing standards.

In summary, federal public health officials plan to rely on the nation's existing influenza surveillance system and enhancements to identify an influenza pandemic. CDC currently collaborates with multiple public health partners, including WHO, to obtain data that provide national and international pictures of influenza activity. Federal public health officials and health care organizations have undertaken several initiatives that are intended to enhance influenza surveillance capabilities. While some of these initiatives are focused more generally on increasing preparedness for bioterrorism and other emerging infectious disease health threats, others were undertaken in preparation for an influenza pandemic. For example, in response to concerns over the past few years about the potential for avian influenza to become the next influenza pandemic, CDC implemented an initiative in cooperation with WHO to improve influenza surveillance in Asia. CDC has also implemented initiatives to improve the communications systems it uses to collect and disseminate surveillance information. In addition, CDC, USDA, and FDA have made efforts to enhance their coordination of surveillance efforts for diseases that arise in animals and can be transferred to humans, such as SARS and certain strains of influenza with the potential to become pandemic.

While public health officials have undertaken several initiatives to enhance influenza surveillance capabilities, challenges remain with regard to other aspects of preparedness for and response to an influenza pandemic. In particular, HHS has not finalized planning for an influenza pandemic. In 2000, we recommended that HHS complete the national plan for responding to an influenza pandemic, but the plan has been in draft format since August 2004. Absent a completed federal plan, key questions about the federal role in the purchase, distribution, and administration of vaccines and antiviral drugs during a pandemic remain unanswered. Other challenges with regard to preparedness for and response to an influenza pandemic exist across the public and private sectors, including challenges in ensuring an adequate and timely influenza vaccine and antiviral supply; addressing regulatory, privacy, and procedural issues surrounding measures to control the spread of disease, for example, across national borders; and resolving issues related to an insufficient hospital and health workforce capacity for responding to a large-scale outbreak such as an influenza pandemic.

---

[5] Disease surveillance is the process of reporting, collecting, analyzing, and exchanging information related to cases of infectious diseases.

[6] See GAO, *Emerging Infectious Diseases: Review of State and Federal Disease Surveillance Efforts,* GAO-04-877 (Washington, D.C.: Sept. 30, 2004).

[7] See "Related GAO Products" at the end of this testimony for a list of our earlier work related to emerging infectious diseases and influenza pandemic planning.

[8] These states—California, Colorado, Indiana, Louisiana, Minnesota, New York, Pennsylvania, Tennessee, Texas, Washington, and Wisconsin—were selected based on their participation in CDC's Emerging Infections Program, each state's most recent infectious disease outbreak, and their geographic location.

BACKGROUND

To be prepared for major public health threats such as an influenza pandemic, public health agencies need several basic capabilities, including disease surveillance systems. Specifically, to detect cases of pandemic influenza, especially before they develop into widespread outbreaks, local, state, and federal public health officials as well as international organizations collect, analyze, and share information related to cases of the disease. When effective, surveillance can facilitate timely action to control outbreaks and promote informed allocation of resources to meet changing disease conditions.

Influenza

Influenza is more severe than some other viral respiratory infections, such as the common cold. Most people who get influenza recover completely in 1 to 2 weeks, but some develop serious and potentially life-threatening medical complications, such as pneumonia. People aged 65 and older, people of any age with chronic medical conditions, children younger than 2 years, and pregnant women are more likely than other people to develop severe complications from influenza. Influenza and pneumonia rank as the fifth leading cause of death among persons aged 65 and older.

Influenza viruses undergo minor but continuous genetic changes from year to year. Almost every year, an influenza virus causes acute respiratory disease in epidemic proportions somewhere in the world. Vaccination is the primary method for preventing influenza and its more severe complications. Influenza vaccine is produced and administered annually to provide protection against particular influenza strains expected to be prevalent that year. Influenza vaccine takes several months to produce. Deciding which viral strains to include in the annual influenza vaccine depends on data collected from domestic and international surveillance systems that identify prevalent strains and characterize their effect on human health. FDA decides which strains to include in the vaccine and also licenses and regulates the manufacturers that produce the vaccine.[9] HHS has limited authority, however, to directly control influenza vaccine production and distribution.[10]

FDA has approved four antiviral medications (amantadine, rimantadine, oseltamivir, and zanamivir) for prevention and treatment of influenza. However, influenza virus strains can become resistant to one or more of these drugs, and so they may not always be effective.

Disease Surveillance and Response

In the United States, responsibility for disease surveillance is shared—involving health care providers; more than 3,000 local health departments, including county, city, and tribal health departments; 59 state and territorial health departments; more than 180,000 public and private laboratories; and public health officials from multiple federal departments and agencies.

States, through the use of their state and local health departments, have principal responsibility for protecting the public's health and therefore take the lead in conducting disease surveillance and supporting response efforts. According to the Institute of Medicine (IOM), most states require health care providers to report any unusual illnesses or deaths—especially those for which a cause cannot be readily established—to their local and/or state health department.[11] Generally, local health departments are responsible for conducting initial investigations into reports of infectious diseases. Laboratory personnel test clinical and environmental samples for possible exposures and identification of illnesses. Epidemiologists in health departments use disease surveillance systems to detect clusters of suspicious symptoms or diseases in order to facilitate early detection and treatment. Local and state health departments monitor disease trends. Local health departments are also responsible for sharing information they obtain from providers or other sources with their state departments of health. State health departments are responsible for collecting surveillance information—which they share on a voluntary basis with CDC and others—from across their state and for coordinating investigations and response efforts.

---

[9] FDA decides which strains to include in the annual influenza vaccine based on the recommendations of its Vaccines and Related Biological Products Advisory Committee.

[10] Under the Federal, Food, Drug and Cosmetic Act, FDA ensures compliance with good manufacturing practices and has limited authority to regulate the resale of prescription drugs, including influenza vaccine, that have been purchased by health care entities, such as public or private hospitals. The term "health care entity" does not include wholesale distributors. This authority would not extend to resale of the vaccine for emergency medical reasons. CDC also has a role in encouraging appropriate public health actions.

[11] The requirement to report clinically anomalous symptoms is particularly important for the detection of emerging infectious diseases, many of which may be unfamiliar to health care providers.

Public health officials provide needed information to the clinical community and the public.

At the federal level, several departments and agencies are involved in disease surveillance and response. For example,

- HHS has primary responsibility for coordinating the nation's response to public health emergencies. As part of its mission, the department has a role in planning to prepare for and respond to an influenza pandemic. One action the department has taken is the development of a draft national pandemic influenza plan, titled "Pandemic Influenza Preparedness and Response Plan."
- CDC is charged with protecting the nation's public health by directing efforts to prevent and control diseases and responding to public health emergencies. It has primary responsibility for conducting national disease surveillance and developing epidemiological and laboratory tools to enhance disease surveillance. CDC also provides an array of technical and financial support for state infectious disease surveillance efforts. In addition, CDC participates in international disease and laboratory surveillance sponsored by WHO.
- FDA is responsible for ensuring that new vaccines and drugs are safe and effective and for conducting research on diagnostic tools and treatment of disease outbreaks. The agency also regulates and licenses vaccines and antiviral agents through the Center for Biologics Evaluation and Research and the Center for Drug Evaluation and Research, respectively. FDA also develops influenza viral reference strains and reagents and makes them available to manufacturers for vaccine development and evaluation.
- The Department of Defense (DOD) contributes to global disease surveillance, training, research, and response to emerging infectious disease threats. DOD maintains the DOD Influenza Surveillance Program, a laboratory-based surveillance program. DOD maintains multiple sites throughout the world that serve as sentinels for disease outbreaks, where it collects and analyzes viral specimens.
- The Department of Agriculture (USDA) is responsible for protecting and improving the health and marketability of animals and animal products by preventing, controlling, and eliminating animal diseases. USDA undertakes disease surveillance and response activities to protect U.S. livestock, ensure the safety of international trade, and contribute to the national zoonotic disease [12] surveillance effort.

The United States is a member of WHO, which is responsible for coordinating international disease surveillance and response efforts. An agency of the United Nations, WHO administers the International Health Regulations, which outline WHO's role and the responsibility of member countries and regions in preventing the global spread of infectious diseases. WHO also helps marshal resources from its members to control outbreaks within individual countries or regions. In addition, WHO works with national governments to improve their surveillance capacities through—for example—assessing and redesigning national surveillance strategies, offering training in epidemiologic and laboratory techniques, and emphasizing more efficient communication systems.

EXISTING INFLUENZA SURVEILLANCE SYSTEM AND ENHANCEMENTS WOULD BE USED TO
IDENTIFY AN INFLUENZA PANDEMIC

Surveillance is a key component in planning for an influenza pandemic, and federal public health officials plan to rely on the nation's existing annual influenza surveillance system and enhancements to identify an influenza pandemic. Federal public health officials have undertaken several initiatives that are intended to enhance influenza surveillance capabilities. These initiatives have been undertaken both through programs specific to influenza as well as through programs focused more generally on increasing preparedness for bioterrorism and other emerging infectious disease health threats. Federal officials have implemented and expanded syndromic surveillance systems [13] in order to detect outbreaks more quickly, but there are concerns that these systems are costly to run and still largely untested. Federal officials have also implemented initiatives designed to improve public health communica-

---

[12] Zoonotic diseases are those diseases that are transmitted from animals to humans.

[13] Many syndromic surveillance systems currently in use in the United States were developed in response to the September 11, 2001, attacks on the World Trade Center and Pentagon and to the anthrax outbreaks that occurred shortly afterwards. The fundamental objective of syndromic surveillance is to identify illness clusters early, before diagnoses are confirmed and reported to public health agencies.

tions and have undertaken initiatives intended to improve the coordination of zoonotic surveillance efforts.

Systems Are in Place to Routinely Monitor for Influenza

Current U.S. surveillance for identifying annual influenza outbreaks as well as an influenza pandemic involves multiple public health partners at all levels of government and relies on several data sources. At the federal level, CDC's Influenza Branch leads the national influenza surveillance effort, monitoring disease and viral trends using data submitted each week from October through May. These surveillance data are collected at the local and state levels and voluntarily submitted to CDC. Data submitted on influenza activity in the United States include data from more than 120 laboratories and 2,000 health care providers and mortality reports from 122 cities. In addition, influenza data are collected from all 50 state health departments and the health departments in the District of Columbia and New York City. CDC also receives data that are specifically focused on influenza in pediatric patients. When the data are used collectively, they provide a national picture of influenza activity. Specifically, they allow CDC to (1) identify when and where influenza activity is occurring, (2) determine what strains of the influenza virus are in circulation, (3) detect changes in the influenza virus, (4) monitor flu-related illnesses, and (5) measure the impact influenza is having on deaths in the United States.

DOD also plays a role in national and international influenza surveillance. Specifically, DOD's Influenza Surveillance Program, under the direction of the Air Force, collects viral specimens from its active duty personnel and their dependents at military facilities around the world. DOD's program also sends specimens to CDC for further analysis and contributes to the determination of which viral strains FDA includes in the nation's annual influenza vaccine. Internationally, DOD provides viral specimens to WHO and assists in identifying emerging influenza strains.

In countries throughout the world, infectious disease surveillance is a national responsibility, but WHO assists its members' efforts through its Global Influenza Surveillance Network. WHO's Network is composed of 112 institutions, called National Influenza Centres, from 83 countries. Collectively, these Centres monitor influenza activity and annually gather more than 175,000 viral specimens for analysis from patients with influenza-like illnesses throughout the world. Selected influenza isolates—an estimated 2,000 viruses—may also be sent to one of four WHO Collaborating Centres [14] for further, more specific genetic analysis. The additional analysis conducted by the WHO Collaborating Centers is used for the annual WHO recommendations on which strains to include in the influenza vaccine for the northern and southern hemispheres. In addition to making recommendations on the components of the influenza vaccine, this Global Influenza Surveillance Network also serves as a global alert mechanism for the emergence of influenza viruses with pandemic potential.

Federal Agencies Have Undertaken Initiatives to Enhance Influenza Surveillance

CDC has undertaken several initiatives that are intended to enhance influenza surveillance capabilities in preparation for an influenza pandemic. CDC works with its international partners to improve global surveillance for influenza. For example, CDC participates in international disease and laboratory surveillance sponsored by WHO. Also, when concerns were raised over recent influenza seasons that the avian influenza A (H5N1) could become the next influenza pandemic, CDC led a variety of efforts with its international partners to plan for and address threats of increased influenza activity worldwide. For example, CDC worked collaboratively with WHO to conduct investigations of avian influenza A in Vietnam and to provide laboratory testing. CDC also provided training assistance and has implemented an initiative to improve influenza surveillance in Asia.

CDC also supports several domestic initiatives to improve surveillance capabilities for influenza. For example, CDC supports enhanced influenza surveillance activities through its Epidemiology and Laboratory Capacity (ELC) Grants. Established in 1997, this program provides funding to state and local influenza programs. Grants have steadily increased from the first awards in 1997, when less than $100,000 was provided to five states through August 2004, with funding totaling more than $2

---

[14] A WHO Collaborating Centre is a national institution designated by WHO to form part of an international collaborative network that contributes to implementing WHO's program priorities and to strengthening institutional capacity in countries and regions. Collaborating Centre activities include collection and dissemination of information, education and training, and participation in collaborative research developed under WHO's leadership. The four Collaborating Centres that are part of WHO's Global Influenza Surveillance Network are located in the United States, Australia, Japan, and the United Kingdom.

million being given to about 47 states or major metropolitan areas. States and cities receiving ELC-influenza funding are encouraged to achieve three highlighted influenza epidemiology and laboratory surveillance capacities: sentinel physician surveillance, viral isolation and subtyping, and year-round surveillance. Each state targets funding to meet one or more of these three priorities and uses funding for support of improvements that include the assignment or hiring of an influenza coordinator, recruitment of sentinel physicians to collect influenza specimens and report influenza-like illness to the state, laboratory infrastructure enhancements to increase influenza testing capabilities for viral isolation and subtyping, and expansion of influenza surveillance activities to year-round.

In an effort to enhance the ability to detect infectious disease outbreaks, particularly in their early stages, federal funding has supported state efforts to implement numerous syndromic surveillance systems. These systems collect information on syndromes from a variety of sources. For example, the National Retail Data Monitor (NRDM) collects data from retail sources instead of hospitals. As of February 2004,—NRDM collected sales data from about 19,000 stores, including pharmacies, in order to monitor sales patterns in such items as over-the-counter influenza medications for signs of a developing infectious disease outbreak.

CDC is taking steps to enhance its two public health communications systems, the Health Alert Network (HAN)[15] and the Epidemic Information Exchange (Epi-X),[16] which are used in disease surveillance and response efforts. For example, CDC is working to increase the number of HAN participants who receive assistance with their communication capacities. In addition, following reports of human deaths from avian influenza A in Vietnam in August 2004, CDC issued a HAN message reiterating criteria for domestic surveillance, diagnostic evaluation, and infection control precautions. CDC also issued detailed laboratory testing procedures for avian influenza through HAN. Similarly, CDC has expanded Epi-X by giving officials at other federal agencies and departments, such as DOD, the ability to use the system. CDC is also adding users to Epi-X from local health departments, giving access to CDC staff in other countries, and making the system available to Field Epidemiology Training Programs (FETP) located in 21 countries.[17] Finally, CDC is facilitating Epi-X's interface with other data sources by allowing users to access the Global Public Health Intelligence Network (GPHIN), the system that searches Web-based media for information on infectious disease outbreaks worldwide.

In addition to the efforts to enhance communication systems, federal public health officials also have enhanced federal coordination for zoonotic disease surveillance and expanded training programs. According to CDC, nearly 70 percent of emerging infectious disease episodes during the past 10 years have been zoonotic diseases. Moreover, recent outbreaks of human disease caused by avian influenza strains in Asia and Europe highlight the potential for new strains to be introduced into the population. Surveillance for zoonotic diseases requires collaboration between animal and human disease specialists. CDC, USDA, and FDA have made efforts to enhance their coordination of zoonotic disease surveillance. For example, CDC and UDSA are working with two national laboratory associations to add veterinary diagnostic laboratories to the Laboratory Response Network (LRN).[18] As of May 2004, 10 veteri-

---

[15] The Health Alert Network (HAN) is an early-warning and response system operated by CDC that is designed to ensure that state and local health departments as well as other federal agencies and departments have timely access to emerging health information.

[16] The Epidemic Information Exchange (Epi-X) is a secure, Web-based communication system operating in all 50 states. CDC uses this system primarily to share information relevant to disease outbreaks with state and local public health officials and with other federal officials. Epi-X also serves as a forum for routine professional discussions and nonemergency inquiries.

[17] In selected foreign locations, CDC operates international training programs, such as FETP. Through FETP, each year CDC trains approximately 50 to 60 physicians and social scientists in applied public health, integrating disease surveillance, applied research, prevention, and control activities. Graduates of the FETP program serve in their native country and provide links between CDC and their respective ministries of health. CDC officials said that trainees from its international programs have frequently provided important information on disease outbreaks.

[18] To strengthen the nation's capacity to rapidly detect biological and chemical agents that could be used as a terrorist weapon, CDC, in partnership with the Federal Bureau of Investigation and the Association of Public Health Laboratories, created LRN in 1999. According to CDC, LRN leverages the resources of 126 laboratories to maintain an integrated national and international network of laboratories that are fully equipped to respond quickly to acts of chemical or biological terrorism, emerging infectious diseases, and other public health threats and emergencies. The network includes federal, state and local public health, military, and international laboratories, as well as laboratories that specialize in food, environmental, and veterinary testing. LRN laboratories have been used in several public health emergencies. For example, in 2001, a Florida LRN laboratory discovered the presence of *Bacillus anthracis,* the pathogen that causes anthrax, in a clinical specimen it tested.

nary laboratories had been added to LRN, and CDC officials told us that they had plans to add more veterinary laboratories in the future. In addition, CDC officials told us the agency has appointed a staff person whose responsibility, in part, is to assist in finding ways to enhance zoonotic disease coordination efforts among federal agencies and departments and with other organizations. This person is helping CDC develop a working group of officials from CDC, USDA, and FDA to coordinate zoonotic disease surveillance.[19] According to CDC officials, the goal of this working group is to explore ways to link existing surveillance systems to better coordinate and integrate surveillance for wildlife, domestic animal, and human diseases. CDC officials also said that the agency is exploring the feasibility of a pilot project to demonstrate this proposed integrated zoonotic disease surveillance system. In addition, USDA officials told us that they hired 23 wildlife biologists in fall 2003 to coordinate disease surveillance, monitoring, and management activities among USDA, CDC, states, and other federal agencies. While each of these initiatives is intended to enhance the surveillance of zoonotic diseases, each is still in the planning stage or the very early stages of implementation.

USDA also conducts influenza surveillance in domestic animals. Coordination with USDA is important because a pandemic strain is likely to arise from genetic mixing of animal and human influenza viruses. Recent outbreaks in domestic poultry in Asia and Europe associated with cases of human disease highlight the importance of coordinating surveillance activities. Surveillance for influenza viruses in poultry in the United States has increased substantially since the outbreak of highly pathogenic avian influenza (HPAI) in Pennsylvania and surrounding states in 1983 and 1984. However, individual states are generally responsible for the development and implementation of surveillance programs that are consistent with the size and complexity of the resident poultry industry.

DESPITE EFFORTS BY FEDERAL OFFICIALS, CHALLENGES REMAIN REGARDING PREPAREDNESS FOR AND RESPONSE TO AN INFLUENZA PANDEMIC

Challenges regarding the nation's preparedness for and response to an influenza pandemic remain. Specifically, our prior work has found that although CDC participated in an interagency working group that developed the U.S. plan for pandemic preparedness that was posted for public comment in August 2004, as of May 23, 2005, the plan had not been finalized. Further, we found that the draft plan does not address certain critical issues, including how vaccine for an influenza pandemic will be purchased, distributed, and administered; how population groups will be prioritized for vaccination; what quarantine authorities or travel restrictions may need to be invoked; and how federal resources should be deployed. At the state level, we found that most hospitals across the country lack the capacity to respond to large-scale infectious disease outbreaks.

HHS's Pandemic Influenza Plan Remains in Draft and Leaves Many Important Issues Unresolved

In August 2004, HHS released its national pandemic influenza plan for comment. The draft "Pandemic Influenza Preparedness and Response Plan" describes HHS's role in coordinating a national response to an influenza pandemic and provides guidance and tools to promote pandemic preparedness planning and coordination at the federal, state, and local levels, including both the public and the private sectors. However, as of May 23, 2005, this document remained in draft form. Further, although the plan is comprehensive in scope, it leaves many important decisions unresolved about the purchase, distribution, and administration of vaccines. For example, some decisions yet to be made include determining the public- versus private-sector roles in the purchase and distribution of pandemic influenza vaccines; the division of responsibility between the federal government and the states for vaccine distribution; and how population groups will be prioritized and targeted to receive limited supplies of vaccines. Until these key decisions are made, public health officials at all levels may find it difficult to plan for an influenza pandemic, and the timeliness and adequacy of response efforts may be compromised.

The draft plan does not establish a definitive federal role in the purchase and distribution of vaccines during an influenza pandemic. Instead, HHS provides options for vaccine purchase and distribution that include public-sector purchase and distribution of all pandemic influenza vaccine; a mixed public-private system where public-sector supply may be targeted to specific priority groups; and maintenance

---

[19] This working group was created in response to a congressional mandate that the Secretary of Health and Human Services, through FDA and CDC, and USDA, coordinate the surveillance of zoonotic diseases. Public Health Security and Bioterrorism Preparedness and Response Act of 2002, Pub. L. No. 107-188, § 313, 116 Stat. 594, 674 (2002).

of the current largely private system. In its draft plan, HHS does not recommend a specific alternative.

Furthermore, the draft plan delegates to the states responsibility for distribution of vaccine. The lack of a clearly defined federal role in distribution complicates pandemic planning for the states. Furthermore, among the current state pandemic influenza plans, there is no consistency in terms of their procurement and distribution of vaccine and the relative role of the federal government. Approximately half of the states handle procurement and distribution of the annual influenza vaccine through the state health agency. The remainder either operate through a third-party contractor for distribution to providers or use a combination of these two approaches.

Challenges Persist in Ensuring an Adequate and Timely Influenza Vaccine Supply

Challenges persist in ensuring an adequate and timely influenza vaccine supply. The number of producers remains limited, and the potential for manufacturing problems such as those experienced during the 2004-2005 influenza season is still present. When one manufacturer's production is affected, providers who order vaccine from that manufacturer can experience shortages, while providers who receive supplies from another manufacturer may have all the vaccine they need. The allocation plan CDC developed for this past season's shortage was dependent upon voluntary compliance by the private sector and individuals to forgo vaccination. Most annual influenza vaccine distribution and administration are accomplished within the private sector, with relatively small amounts of vaccine purchased and distributed by CDC or by state and local health departments. In the United States, 85 percent of vaccine doses are purchased by the private sector, such as private physicians and pharmacies. HHS has not yet determined how influenza vaccine will be distributed and administered during an influenza pandemic.

There are many issues surrounding the production of influenza vaccine, which will only become exacerbated during an influenza pandemic. Vaccines, which are considered the first line of defense to prevent or reduce influenza-related illness and death, may be unavailable or in short supply. Producing the vaccine is a complex process that involves growing viruses in millions of fertilized chicken eggs. Experience has shown that the vaccine production cycle takes at least 6 to 8 months after a virus strain has been identified, and vaccines for some influenza strains have been difficult to mass-produce, causing further delay. The lengthy process for developing a vaccine may mean that a vaccine would not be available during the initial stages of a pandemic.

Vaccine shortages during the 2004-2005 influenza season have highlighted the fragility of the influenza vaccine market and the need for its expansion and stabilization. Currently only two manufacturers are licensed to sell their vaccine in the United States.[20] Maintaining an influenza vaccine supply is critically important for protecting the public's health and improving our preparedness for an influenza pandemic. As a result, according to CDC officials, the agency plans to alleviate the impact of next year's influenza season by taking aggressive steps to ensure an expanded influenza supply to protect the nation. To this end, the agency's fiscal year 2006 budget request includes an increase of $30 million for CDC to enter into guaranteed purchase contracts with vaccine manufacturers to ensure the production of bulk monovalent influenza vaccine. If supplies fall short, this bulk product can be turned into a finished trivalent influenza vaccine product for annual distribution. If supplies are sufficient, the bulk vaccine can be held until the following year's influenza season and developed into vaccines if the circulating strains remain the same. In addition, according to CDC, this guarantee will help to expand the influenza market by providing an incentive to manufacturers to expand capacity and possibly encourage additional manufacturers to enter the market. In addition, the fiscal year 2006 budget request includes an increase of $20 million to support influenza vaccine purchase activities.

Even if sufficient quantities of the vaccine are produced in time, vaccines against various strains differ in their ability to produce the immune response necessary to provide effective protection against the disease. Studies show that it is uncertain how effective a vaccine will be in preventing or controlling the spread of a pandemic influenza virus.

Challenges Persist in Ensuring an Adequate Supply of Antiviral Drugs

Early in an influenza pandemic, especially before a vaccine is available or during a period of limited vaccine supply, use of antiviral drugs may have a significant effect. Specifically, antiviral drugs can help prevent or mitigate the number of influ-

---

[20] During the 2004-2005 influenza season, the license for a third manufacturer was suspended by British regulatory authorities due to safety concerns with the vaccine.

enza-related deaths until an influenza vaccine becomes available. They can be used against all strains of pandemic influenza and have immediate availability as both a prophylactic to prevent illness and as a treatment if administered within 48 hours of the onset of symptoms. According to HHS, analysis is ongoing to define optimal antiviral use strategies, potential health impacts, and cost-effectiveness of antiviral drugs in the setting of a pandemic.

The United States has a limited supply of influenza antiviral medications stored for an influenza pandemic. HHS officials expect the amount produced will be below demand during a pandemic. This assumption, supported by drug manufacturers, is based on the fact that current production levels of antiviral drugs are set in response to current demand, whereas demand in a pandemic is expected to increase significantly if vaccines are unavailable. In addition, the production of antiviral medications cannot be rapidly expanded and involves a long production process—at least 6 to 9 months. Moreover, sometimes influenza virus strains can become resistant to one or more of the four approved influenza antiviral drugs, and thus the drugs may not always work. For example, the influenza A (H5N1) viruses identified in human patients in Asia in 2004 and 2005 have been resistant to two of the four antiviral drugs, amantadine and rimantadine.

Implementation of Control Measures to Prevent Spread of Pandemic Influenza Present Difficulties

Another challenge in responding to an influenza pandemic involves implementing certain control measures to prevent the spread of the disease. These control measures—case identification and contact tracing, transmission control, and exposure management—are well-established and have proved effective in both health care and community settings.[21] Federal attempts to limit the spread of SARS into the United States by advising passengers who traveled to infected countries faced multiple obstacles. For example, due to airline concerns over authority and privacy, as well as procedural constraints, CDC was unable to obtain passenger contact information it needed to trace travelers. Although HHS has statutory authority to prevent the introduction, transmission, or spread of communicable diseases from foreign countries into the United States,[22] HHS regulations implementing the statute do not specifically provide for HHS to obtain passenger manifests or other passenger contact information from airlines and shipping companies for disease outbreak control purposes.[23]

Most Hospitals Lack the Capacity to Respond to Large-Scale Infectious Disease Outbreaks

A challenge identified during the SARS outbreak that may also affect response efforts during an influenza pandemic is lack of sufficient hospital and workforce capacity. This lack could be exacerbated during an influenza pandemic, compared to other natural disasters, such as a tornado or hurricane, or an intentional release of a bioterrorist agent, because it is likely that a pandemic would result in both widespread and sustained effects.

Public health officials we spoke with said a large-scale outbreak, such as an influenza pandemic, could strain the available capacity of hospitals by requiring the use of entire hospital sections (along with their staff) to be used as isolation facilities. As we have reported earlier, most states lack "surge capacity," that is, the capacity to respond to the large influx of patients that could occur during a large public health emergency.[24] For example, few states reported that they had the capacity to evaluate, diagnose, and treat 500 or more patients involved in a single incident. In addition, few states reported having the capacity to rapidly establish clinics to immunize or provide treatment to large numbers of patients. Moreover, a shortage in workforce could increase during an influenza pandemic because higher disease rates

---

[21] In the United States, the Healthcare Infection Control Practices Advisory Committee, a federal advisory committee made up of 14 infection control experts, develops recommendations and guidelines regarding general infectious disease control measures for CDC. Expert recommendations include (1) case identification and contact tracing, which involves defining what symptoms, laboratory results, and medical histories constitute a positive case in a patient and tracing and tracking individuals who may have been exposed to these patients; (2) transmission control, which involves controlling the transmission of disease-producing microorganisms through use of proper hand hygiene and personal protective equipment, such as masks, gowns, and gloves; and (3) exposure management, which involves separating infected and noninfected individuals.

[22] Section 361 of the Public Health Service Act, 42 U.S.C. § 264.

[23] See 42 C.F.R pts 70 and 71; 21 C.F.R. pts 1240 and 1250.

[24] See GAO, *Public Health Preparedness: Response Capacity Improving, but Much Remains to be Accomplished,* GAO-04-458T (Washington, D.C.: Feb. 12, 2004).

could result in high rates of absenteeism among health care workers who are likely to be at increased risk of exposure and illness.

CONCLUDING OBSERVATIONS

There are a number of systems in place to identify influenza outbreaks abroad, to alert us to a pandemic, and these systems generally appear to be working well. HHS has taken important steps to enhance surveillance and to fund initiatives for preparedness and response, including steps to increase the vaccine supply.

However, important challenges remain in our preparedness to respond, should an influenza pandemic occur in the United States. The steps HHS is taking to address vaccine production capacity and stockpiling of antiviral drugs may not be in place in time to fill the current gaps in preparedness should an influenza pandemic occur in the next several years. As we learned in the 2004-2005 influenza season, problems affecting even a single manufacturer can produce major shortages. Once a pandemic influenza strain is identified, a vaccine will take many months to produce, and our current stockpile of antiviral drugs is insufficient to meet the likely demand. Pandemic influenza would have major impacts on the ability of communities to respond, businesses to function, and public safety to be maintained when communities across the country are simultaneously impacted and hospital capacity is overwhelmed.

Since 2000, we have been urging the department to complete its pandemic plan. A draft plan was issued in August 2004, with a 60-day period for public comment, but as of this week, the plan had not been finalized. It is important for the federal government and the states to work through issues such as how vaccine will be purchased, distributed, and administered, how population groups will be prioritized for vaccination, what quarantine authorities or travel restrictions may need to be invoked, and how federal resources should be deployed before we are in a time of crisis.

Mr. Chairman, this concludes my prepared statement. I would be happy to respond to any questions you or other Members of the Subcommittee may have at this time.

Contact and Staff Acknowledgments

For further information about this testimony, please contact Marcia Crosse at (202) 512-7119. Gloria E. Taylor, Gay Hee Lee, Elizabeth T. Morrison, and Roseanne Price made key contributions to this statement.

RELATED GAO PRODUCTS

Emerging Infectious Diseases: Review of State and Federal Disease Surveillance Efforts. GAO-04-877. Washington, D.C.: September 30, 2004.

Infectious Disease Preparedness: Federal Challenges in Responding to Influenza Outbreaks. GAO-04-1100T. Washington, D.C.: September 28, 2004.

Emerging Infectious Diseases: Asian SARS Outbreak Challenged International and National Responses. GAO-04-564. Washington, D.C.: April 28, 2004.

Public Health Preparedness: Response Capacity Improving, but Much Remains to Be Accomplished. GAO-04-458T. Washington, D.C.: February 12, 2004.

Infectious Diseases: Gaps Remain in Surveillance Capabilities of State and Local Agencies. GAO-03-1176T. Washington, D.C.: September 24, 2003.

Severe Acute Respiratory Syndrome: Established Infectious Disease Control Measures Helped Contain Spread, But a Large-Scale Resurgence May Pose Challenges. GAO-03-1058T. Washington, D.C.: July 30, 2003.

SARS Outbreak: Improvements to Public Health Capacity Are Needed for Responding to Bioterrorism and Emerging Infectious Diseases. GAO-03-769T. Washington, D.C.: May 7, 2003.

Infectious Disease Outbreaks: Bioterrorism Preparedness Efforts Have Improved Public Health Response Capacity, but Gaps Remain. GAO-03-654T. Washington, D.C.: April 9, 2003.

Global Health: Challenges in Improving Infectious Disease Surveillance Systems. GAO-01-722. Washington, D.C.: August 31, 2001.

Flu Vaccine: Steps Are Needed to Better Prepare for Possible Future Shortages. GAO-01-786T. Washington, D.C.: May 30, 2001.

Flu Vaccine: Supply Problems Heighten Need to Ensure Access for High-Risk People. GAO-01-624. Washington, D.C.: May 15, 2001.

Influenza Pandemic: Plan Needed for Federal and State Response. GAO-01-4. Washington, D.C.: October 27, 2000.

West Nile Virus Outbreak: Lessons for Public Health Preparedness. GAO/HEHS-00-180. Washington, D.C.: September 11, 2000.

Global Health: Framework for Infectious Disease Surveillance. GAO/NSIAD-00-205R. Washington, D.C.: July 20, 2000.

Mr. FERGUSON. Thank you very much. Dr. Pavia.

STATEMENT OF ANDREW T. PAVIA

Mr. PAVIA. Yes. Mr. Chairman, members of the committee, thank you very much for inviting the IDSA to make its opinion felt and heard about pandemic influenza. I am Andrew Pavia. I am Chair of the Infectious Diseases Society of America's Taskforce on Pandemic Influenza and also professor of Pediatric Infectious Disease and chief at the University of Utah.

IDSA, so that you know, represents over 8,000 infectious disease experts, including all three of the members of the first panel and soon to be Mr. Green's daughter, who work in taking care of patients with the most severe infectious disease and conducting laboratory research and in public health. And let me be very clear that although this is a mixed panel, I am speaking on behalf of the physicians, our patients, and the public health.

Like everyone else who has spoken today, IDSA believes that the next pandemic is inevitable, but more importantly, we believe that the evidence suggests that it may be imminent. We don't know whether H5N1, Avian Flu, will be the next pandemic strain. We don't know how severe the next pandemic will be. We do know, however, that it will occur, and we know that the severity is going to be somewhere between severe and catastrophic.

For all that you have heard it is hard to overemphasize or exaggerate the potential impact of a pandemic. You heard the figures for CDC's estimate of the mortality and impact of a moderate pandemic. Their same estimates suggest that if we have a pandemic with a virus that has the severity equivalent to 1918, that it would result in between .9 and 2.2 million deaths and four to ten million hospitalizations. Now, imagine the economic impact of paying for four to ten million hospitalizations. And I am going to come back to the economics a little bit because some of the countermeasures require sufficient funding.

As we think about the economic impact, these figures have not been fully worked out, but as was pointed out in yesterday's "Wall Street Journal" editorial and by several analysts, it is likely that even a mild pandemic would bring global economies to a halt, it would devastate the agriculture, and it would probably pose a grave threat to national security. If you think about the costs that we have seen from relatively mild epidemics before, consider SARS. Fewer than 8,000 people were sickened and about 800 died, and yet the estimate is that for countries affected in Southeast Asia, the cost ranged between .2 and 1.8 percent of their GDP. The city of Toronto lost over $1 billion alone. These are the kind of figures that you need to think about when you think about the cost of the countermeasures.

Now, I want to be very clear that pandemic influenza has received a great deal of attention from the government, from Congress, and we are very grateful. And you have heard a great deal about what is being done at the Federal Government level in the earlier panel. And I want to point out that NVPO in particular has taken a leadership position in this, and that is very, very important. However, as of today, the IDSA believes that the United States is woefully unprepared for a pandemic that might occur in the next few years.

We have many recommendations in our written testimony, and I am going to focus my remaining comments on areas where scientists alone can't deal with the problem, and it requires activity by policymakers. The first and foremost is adequate funding of our public health efforts. And IDSA has recommended not only restoring the cuts in the CDC budget, but appropriate increases. And I think that that goes across the board for our public health infrastructure.

Many have pointed out the fragility of our vaccine supply as highlighted by the events of last fall. But I think what we haven't emphasized is that the capacity to produce vaccine is really the critical issue. And the same holds true for antivirals. It is assumed by most experts in the event of a crisis we are going to be totally dependent on what can be produced domestically. And if we look at the capacity to produce vaccine domestically, we can make between 60 and 70 million doses of trivalent vaccine. That means that perhaps with a monovalent vaccine we could produce 180 million doses after a lag time of about 6 months and a year to produce that 180 million doses. The estimate is we would need two doses for every man, woman, and child in the United States, or 600 million doses. Clearly, we are either going to have to dramatically increase the capacity to produce vaccine or the efficiency with which it can be produced or the number of people we can immunize with a given amount of vaccine.

To that end a great deal of progress has been made. You have heard from HHS and from NIH about the beginnings of programs to fund improvements in the efficacy of vaccine production and ways to look at antigen-sparing techniques that would use less vaccine. I think that if we look at it objectively, when my question, whether it is too little and whether it might be too late, but in order to have a robust response we need more capacity to produce vaccine domestically. That means we need a dramatically greater use of vaccine year-in, year-out. And to that end I think that Congress can have a role in increasing incentives for companies to enter the vaccine market so that we have a more diverse production and that we use more vaccine in every year.

Now, I think it is also worth pointing out that every dollar we spend on countermeasures for pandemic flu—I promise this isn't Avian Influenza—no coughing—that every dollar we spend on pandemic flu will yield an annual benefit in preventing lives lost for our yearly flu epidemics.

I want to turn our attention for a moment to stockpile. That has come up before. And I have to respectfully disagree with what Dr. Gerberding said earlier. An expert panel that is advising the National Vaccine Advisory Committee that will go into the pandemic plan feels that in the first 6 months of an epidemic the use of antivirals will be a major tool that we have, if not the only tool, to decrease morbidity and mortality and to allow the vital functions of government and of the healthcare system to continue.

To that end we need to have an adequate stockpile. IDSA's leadership, perhaps as a strawman, has suggested that we purchase enough antivirals to treat 50 percent of the United States population. Now, we know that our allies in Europe have planned on purchasing enough to treat between 20 and 25 percent. All of these numbers are crudely derived. There are more scientific efforts underway to figure out what the actual need would be. But it will likely range between 60 million and 150 million doses. The 2.3 million doses we have in the U.S. stockpile currently are clearly inadequate.

The cost of purchasing antivirals for the stockpile is going to be considerable. It can't be redirected from existing health resources. It can't be redirected from within HHS. And it is going to require considerable outside appropriation. But as I hope I have made clear, the costs of not doing something will far exceed the cost of developing a stockpile.

Another issue that is important is that the entire production of oseltamivir or Tamiflu, as of today, is made in Switzerland. And as I mentioned earlier, it may not be available to the United States in a time of crisis.

A question was asked about indemnification earlier. We have learned from past experiences that in 1976 that the manufacturers were reluctant to release vaccine in the absence of liability productions. We learned 2 years ago in the attempts to provide small pox immunization that hospitals and providers were reluctant to give small pox vaccine without having some form of indemnification against problems that arose.

And a third problem is how are we going to compensate people who might be injured by an experimental vaccine? Clearly, we need to have some sort of vaccine injury compensation coverage for a pandemic vaccine.

Mr. FERGUSON. Dr. Pavia, I am just going to ask you to summarize, please.

Mr. PAVIA. Very good. I am going to stop my comments there. You can tell that I am a professor and used to having the floor. Only slightly worse, I suppose, than being a member. But thank you very much for having us and for the attention and the expertise that you bring today.

[The prepared statement of Andrew T. Pavia follows:]

PREPARED STATEMENT OF ANDREW T. PAVIA, INFECTIOUS DISEASES SOCIETY OF AMERICA

Chairman Deal, Ranking Member Brown, and Members of the House Energy and Commerce Health Subcommittee, thank you for inviting the Infectious Diseases Society of America (IDSA) to present our views on the U.S. preparedness for pandemic influenza and to allow us to share with you our perspective on activities needed to strengthen the nation's current approach. I am Dr. Andrew T. Pavia, chair of IDSA's Task Force on Pandemic Influenza, and professor and chief of the Division of Pediatric Infectious Diseases at the University of Utah Health Sciences Center and Primary Children's Hospital.

IDSA represents nearly 8,000 infectious disease (ID) experts, many of whom administer the flu vaccine to patients, treat life-threatening complications of influenza, conduct vaccine and antiviral research, and implement influenza surveillance activities and other important influenza public health programs at the local, state, and federal levels. Let me be very clear from the onset: Although we are speaking on the same panel as our industry colleagues, our testimony is provided strictly for the good of public health and the patients whom we treat. IDSA is not here on behalf of the pharmaceutical or biotechnology industries nor is our advocacy financed in any way by industry.

IDSA IS SERIOUSLY CONCERNED ABOUT THE NEXT INFLUENZA PANDEMIC

Like our colleagues in federal government, we believe that the next influenza pandemic is imminent. These predictions are primarily based upon the historic intervals between outbreaks as well as the increased spread and ominous behavior of the H5N1 avian influenza virus, which now is endemic among birds in much of Asia. We are very concerned that the H5N1 avian virus has shown the ability to mutate and has become capable of infecting mammals, including pigs, tigers, cats, and humans as well as birds. At least 97 confirmed human cases of H5N1 infections have been documented by the World Health Organization (WHO) since January 2004 with 53 deaths. A recent WHO consultants meeting found evidence of further mutation and a suggestion that person-to-person transmission might be occurring in Northern Vietnam. Should the virus become readily transmissible from human to human, the disease could easily spread beyond Asia's borders and initiate a global pandemic. The U.S. population has no immunity and therefore no protection against this deadly virus. Implications of Pandemic Influenza for the United States

The impact of a pandemic influenza outbreak cannot be overemphasized. During the past century, influenza pandemics occurred in 1918, 1957, and 1968, with significant morbidity and mortality in both high-risk and healthy children and adults. These outbreaks cost the lives of hundreds of thousands of Americans. Historians now estimate that between 50 million and 100 million people died as a result of the 1918 influenza pandemic alone. More than half a million Americans died, many of them young adults in the prime of life. Although the 1956 and 1968 pandemics were not as severe, the current mortality rate among patients with H5N1 influenza is more than 50 percent compared with 2.5 to 5 percent for the disastrous 1918 pandemic virus. The Centers for Disease Control and Prevention (CDC) has estimated that a pandemic as severe as the 1918 pandemic would cause between 0.9 and 2.2 million deaths and 4 million to 10 million hospitalizations in the United States.

The next pandemic will cause much economic and social chaos. There will be a dramatic impact on the U.S. and global economies, and potentially on civil order and international security. Consider the billions of dollars of economic impact of the severe acute respiratory syndrome (SARS) epidemic. SARS was trivial in size and scope compared with even a modest flu pandemic.

UNITED STATES IS NOT ADEQUATELY PREPARED

Congress and the Administration have begun to realize the real threat that influenza poses to the United States as evident by the allocation of additional monies for influenza activities in recent years. The Administration has proposed an additional $120 million for influenza preparedness activities in the fiscal year 2006 budget to further strengthen pandemic influenza preparedness efforts. While welcome, this is a small investment. Additionally, the Department of Health and Human Services (HHS) recently proposed a thoughtful and scientifically based draft pandemic preparedness and response plan that lays out public health measures to counter a sudden worldwide influenza epidemic. IDSA has provided extensive comments on the plan and currently is participating on an HHS workgroup to develop specific policies and improve preparedness. CDC has worked to strengthen its scientific and epidemiologic capacity to respond. The National Institutes of Health (NIH) has begun efforts to develop vaccine for avian influenza and has increased support for other basic research.

IDSA recognizes and appreciates the increasing level of federal support for U.S. preparedness efforts. However, IDSA agrees with the Institute of Medicine and virtually all experts who have concluded that the United States is at present woefully unprepared to respond to the next flu pandemic.

Two promising strategies can decrease the impact of a flu pandemic. Vaccination is the primary strategy to prevent influenza during normal years and during a pandemic. The recent shortage of flu vaccine highlights the fragility of our nation's vaccine supply. We clearly need a greater capacity to produce vaccine. This means we must attract more vaccine manufacturers to produce influenza vaccine within our borders. It has been estimated that vaccinating the U.S. population against a pandemic flu strain might require 600 million doses of vaccine (two doses for each person might be needed). Even in a normal year, only 50 million to 60 million doses of vaccine can be manufactured in the United States. Counting doses of vaccine imported from abroad, about 90 million doses are used. In the best case, it will take four to six months to begin to produce a pandemic influenza vaccine. Unfortunately, only three influenza vaccine manufacturers currently produce flu vaccines for the U.S. market; only one of them produces its vaccine within the United States.

Antiviral drugs would be the only available agents for treatment and prevention in the early phase of a pandemic. However, adequate supplies will not be available unless decisive action is taken. Global production of these agents is modest. If antivirals are to be available in an emergency they would need to be stockpiled in advance.

Strengthening our pandemic influenza preparedness activities also will provide significant benefits during the typical "interpandemic" flu season when 36,000 American lives are lost and 200,000 are hospitalized each year. The same cannot be said for preparedness activities for intentional biological emergencies such as smallpox, which does not exist in nature, or anthrax, which is an extremely rare disease.

POTENTIAL LEGISLATIVE AND ADMINISTRATIVE SOLUTIONS

Considering the significance of the threat, IDSA has identified the following short and long term strategies to strengthen the U.S. level of preparedness and response to both interpandemic and pandemic influenza.

Secure vaccine and antiviral supplies.

Adequate supplies of antivirals and if possible vaccine, need to be in place before a pandemic strikes, along with a plan to distribute them. More must be done to bring additional manufacturers into the vaccine business, particularly to develop domestic based companies so that the United States is not dependent on foreign suppliers. Increased use of vaccine during interpandemic years is needed to increase the manufacturing capacity. Without this strengthened capacity, we will be unable to meet the high demand that will occur during an influenza pandemic.

Stockpiles of antiviral drugs are also essential. IDSA has proposed a stockpile of antivirals sufficient to treat 50 percent of the U.S. population. This stockpile will help to reduce mortality and allow vital services such as medical care and emergency services to continue. Clearly, the current stockpile, which could treat less than 2 percent of the U.S. population, is inadequate. The cost of developing an adequate stockpile cannot be paid for by shifting funds within HHS agencies; it will require a separate appropriation. Given the enormous burden of illness and death anticipated in a pandemic, however, this investment promises an excellent return. In addition, the entire production capacity for oseltamivir is located in Switzerland. As with influenza vaccines, IDSA fully supports the development of antiviral production capacities within the United States.

It is essential that we develop a specific strategy to distribute antiviral drugs and vaccines to states, local health departments, and points-of-care. We support the effort currently underway by the Pandemic Influenza Working Group of the National Vaccine Advisory Committee (NVAC) to provide detailed estimates of the priorities for use of antivirals and the amount of drug needed to reach different target groups. This will provide more precise estimates of the size and cost of a stockpile needed to provide a specific level of benefit.

Advance Research and Development of Antivirals and Vaccines.

Current manufacturing of influenza vaccine depends on egg-based technology that is 60 years old. It imposes limits on the ability to ramp up production and to work with strains that are lethal to eggs. Research and development of newer vaccines is vital. NIH has recently outlined funding for work on cell-culture based vaccine and for antigen-sparing approaches. These are vital efforts and should be accelerated. Equal attention needs to be paid to our ability to rapidly and safely license new technologies to produce new vaccines for widespread use. Truly innovative vaccines could be developed that do not need to be redesigned each year. Investment in this research could be extremely important but will take many years to realize a benefit.

Research also is needed to develop new antivirals with anti-influenza activity. We are currently dependent on a single agent, oseltamavir (also known as Tamiflu, an antiviral produced by Roche Pharmaceuticals). In the event H5N1 becomes a pandemic strain, this vulnerability will be dangerous.

Create tax incentives for U.S. vaccine and antiviral manufacturers.

The United States does not have the manufacturing capacity to produce enough vaccine and antivirals to meet its needs in a pandemic. Tax credits should be offered to encourage companies to build new manufacturing facilities in this country so that the United States is not dependent on foreign suppliers. Tax incentives and patent extensions should be available for companies that conduct research and develop new anti-flu therapies.

Guarantee a market for influenza vaccines.

Most pharmaceutical companies have left the vaccine business because demand is extremely unpredictable. Even last season, when there was a severe shortage of vaccine, millions of doses of flu vaccine went unused. To secure vaccine supplies for future influenza outbreaks, the government needs to guarantee it will buy a set amount of vaccine each season, and buy back a percentage of unsold vaccine at the end of each season.

The Centers for Medicare and Medicaid Services (CMS) also has a critical role to play. The recent increase in the Medicare reimbursement for administration of flu vaccine, although long overdue, was a positive step. However, the current system still places physicians at financial risk, which may have consequences for patient access to vaccine. Physicians must purchase vaccine annually in advance of the flu season. Unused vaccine is then discarded at the end of the flu season. Physicians are not compensated for the unused product, which, of course, may make them less inclined to purchase vaccine in advance in future years. As all Medicare beneficiaries should receive annual influenza vaccine, CMS should consider how to purchase enough vaccine for Medicare patients in a manner that does not place physicians at risk.

Strengthen liability protection during emergency outbreak response.

In case of a declared influenza emergency, it will be vital to immunize and treat large numbers of people. Even rare adverse reactions following vaccination and treatment would become more common when hundreds of millions are treated, and accelerated approval of new vaccines and treatments might not uncover all rare adverse events. Health care workers and medical facilities administering vaccines or treatments, as well as the companies that make them, should be protected from lawsuits stemming from adverse events so long as they follow standard medical and manufacturing procedures. A compensation fund similar in structure to the Vaccine Injury Compensation Fund should be established to cover the medical costs and lost earnings of anyone who develops complications due to vaccination or treatment.

Improve coordination, communication, and planning.

Many federal, state, and local agencies have vital roles in preparedness, planning, and response. HHS should develop a detailed plan to coordinate pandemic response at all levels, from local to national to international, including links between federal authorities and clinicians throughout the country. HHS should also define CDC as the coordinating authority within the department. Moreover, there needs to be a clear ability to coordinate efforts between departments, including not only HHS, but also Defense, Agriculture (USDA), Homeland Security, and State.

Require health care workers to be vaccinated.

Unfortunately, health care workers caring for sick people often spread patients' infections. In 2002, only 36 percent of U.S. health care workers received influenza vaccine. To improve patient safety, prevent unnecessary deaths and disease, and provide an example to patients, we believe that annual flu vaccination should be required for all health care workers who have contact with patients, with options to waive vaccination after signing an appropriate waiver.

Strengthen education.

Health care workers and the public need to better understand the seriousness and potential impact of an influenza pandemic, as well as how to prevent and treat it.

Commit to international pandemic preparedness.

A coordinated international effort is vital. The United States should work with other countries, particularly those most vulnerable, on plans to ensure that they have sufficient antiviral and vaccine supplies to protect their populations.

Strengthen the response of federal agencies.

The Food and Drug Administration should "fast-track" vaccine and antiviral review, and streamline regulation of the manufacturing process. Congress should increase the CDC's budget for global surveillance to detect influenza strains with pandemic potential. The NIH budget also should be increased for research to identify and evaluate new methods to accelerate vaccine research and development. USDA should develop a plan for culling poultry or other livestock and compensating farmers in the event of a pandemic, if necessary.

CONCLUSION

The United States remains unprepared for pandemic influenza that could kill millions of Americans over a short period of time with little warning. We may not have much time. The United States needs a rational, integrated, and comprehensive plan that will ensure an effective response. We also need a better-coordinated approach, both domestically and globally. If IDSA's recommendations are implemented, our nation will be better prepared for both the next pandemic and for influenza outbreaks that occur every year. As Winston Churchill said: "It is not enough to say, 'We are doing our best.' You have got to succeed in doing what is necessary."

IDSA appreciates the opportunity to testify before the House Energy and Commerce Health Subcommittee today. We look forward to working with you in the coming months to develop federal legislation needed to strengthen U.S. efforts to prepare for the next influenza pandemic.

Thank you. I will be happy to answer any questions.

Mr. FERGUSON. You are definitely in the right room. Mr. Hosbach.

STATEMENT OF PHILLIP HOSBACH

Mr. HOSBACH. Mr. Chairman, members of the committee, I would like to thank you for the opportunity to speak with you today and more importantly, for holding this critically important hearing.

Sanofi pasteur is committed to working with the Federal Government to develop a safe and effective pandemic vaccine to protect the American public. Today I would like to outline four necessary steps to develop and administer a pandemic influenza vaccine.

Sanofi pasteur is the world's largest influenza vaccine manufacturer. We produce vaccines against more than 20 diseases. Worldwide we distribute almost one billion doses of vaccine annually. Our U.S. operations are located in Swiftwater, Pennsylvania where influenza vaccine has been produced for more than 30 years. Approximately 95 percent of that influenza vaccine that is made in Swiftwater is used exclusively in the United States.

In the past decade sanofi pasteur has steadily increased U.S. production of influenza vaccine. Last year we produced 58 million doses. We are in the final design stages of our influenza vaccine facility expansion and we also recently invested in a new expanded filling and packaging facility. Both of these projects will significantly expand our U.S. influenza vaccine production and capacity.

As most of you know, vaccines by their very nature are challenging to develop, produce, and distribute. We believe the expertise of vaccine manufacturers, particularly those with a track record in influenza vaccine production and distribution should be utilized early in the planning process.

The enormous public health threat posed by a pandemic prompted sanofi pasteur to take specific steps for a comprehensive pandemic strategy, including the formation of a global working group to examine preparedness, production, distribution, and communication issues. We have cooperated with HHS exchanging ideas on how best to prepare for and respond to a pandemic.

In addition, we entered into several contracts with the Federal Government. We received two H5N1 pandemic influenza vaccine contracts, as mentioned by Dr. Fauci. In accordance with these agreements, we delivered 8,000 investigational doses of H5N1 vaccine to NIH for the clinical trials that have already started. We also produced two million H5N1 bulk doses at large scale.

Sanofi pasteur also received a contract to establish and maintain flocks of egg-laying hens on a year-round basis. As you know, eggs are utilized early in the stages of vaccine production, and prior to this agreement, were only available on a seasonal basis. Finally, sanofi pasteur was awarded a contract to speed development of a cell culture influenza vaccine in the United States.

Mr. Chairman, we are encouraged by the increased attention pandemic planning is receiving from the government, industry, international agencies, and key stakeholders. However, the failure to address critical challenges could aversely affect our ability to respond to a pandemic. I would like to outline four steps necessary to develop and administer a pandemic influenza vaccine.

First, we need to steadily increase inter-pandemic immunization rates. Manufacturers will produce additional vaccine to meet predicatble demand. Steady and sustained increase in inter-pandemic demand will give manufacturers the confidence to continue expansion plans and new companies an incentive to enter the marketplace. To achieve this all key stakeholders need to work together to encourage higher influenza immunization rates. As a Nation, we have never immunized more than 85 million people in any given year. We can and must do better.

Second, we need to ensure proper combination of private and public sector distribution of a vaccine in a pandemic. While it will be important to establish mechanisms for mass immunizations in public clinics, private physicians' offices will also play a key role in a pandemic. During a typical influenza season, the private sector distributes over 85 percent of the Nation's supply. The private market itself provides maximum flexibility in vaccine distribution.

Last year's influenza vaccine shortage illustrated sanofi pasteur's unique expertise in shipping product to any U.S. location within 24 to 48 hours. We ship vaccines to any users in accordance with the CDC's recommendations and distribution plan. Our unprecedented collaboration with the CDC underscores our commitment to America's public health.

Third, vaccine liability protection is another critical issue in pandemic preparedness. A special compensation liability protection program will need to be established similar to the 1976 Swine Flu and 2002 small pox models. The pandemic liability program should be distinct and separate from the existing Vaccine Injury Compensation Program and should focus exclusively on a monovalent influenza vaccine. Failure to offer liability protection could have profound implications for the development, testing, and subsequent licensure and administration of doses of vaccine. It is important to address liability before a health emergency arises. We urge Congress to establish liability protections as strong as those afforded providers of small pox vaccine under the Homeland Security Act of 2002. Strong and effective vaccine liability provisions ensure that manufacturers can bring a pandemic vaccine to market as quickly as possible.

Finally, CDC must continue to build a pediatric vaccine stockpile. I think many of the members of the panel have already spoken about that. Let me reiterate, when an influenza pandemic strikes the United States, sanofi pasteur will have to shift personnel and other resources away from routine vaccine production to optimize production of a monovalent pandemic influenza vaccine. Congress has appropriated funds to establish stockpiles of routine childhood vaccines to be used in case of a disruption in supply, but most funds remain unused. And I won't go into any further detail because I think we have further details there.

But finally, sanofi pasteur is committed to protecting America's public health in the fight against influenza through immunization. We want to commend Congress and the administration for dedicating time and resources to this critical area. Thank you.

[The prepared statement of Phillip Hosbach follows:]

PREPARED STATEMENT OF PHILIP HOSBACH, VICE PRESIDENT, IMMUNIZATION POLICY AND GOVERNMENT AFFAIRS, SANOFI PASTEUR

On behalf of sanofi pasteur, thank you for the opportunity to testify today before the Energy and Commerce Subcommittee on Health. Sanofi pasteur is committed to working with the federal government to develop a safe and effective vaccine to protect the American public in the event of an influenza pandemic. Our common goal is to provide sufficient vaccine for 300 million Americans within the first 12- to 18-month period of a pandemic, and we welcome the chance to provide the committee with our perspective on this important public health issue.

Sanofi pasteur, the world's largest influenza vaccine manufacturer, also manufactures vaccines against more than 20 different diseases. Worldwide, we produce almost 1 billion doses of vaccines annually. The company, which employs more than 9,000 employees worldwide, is headquartered in Lyon, France. Sanofi pasteur's US operations are located in the Pocono Mountains in Swiftwater, Pa., at a site where vaccine has been produced for more than 100 years. Influenza vaccine has been produced in this facility for more than 30 years and 95% of this vaccine is used exclusively to supply the United States. Sanofi pasteur also has an influenza vaccine production facility in France that supplies other markets.

During the past decade, sanofi pasteur has reliably and consistently increased production of influenza vaccine in the US. Last year, we produced 58 million doses for the US market. We continue to expand our vaccine manufacturing capacity in Pennsylvania and have embarked on the largest infrastructure investment in the company's history, spending almost $80 million to build a new formulation and filling facility. We are also in the final design phases of our influenza vaccine facility expansion, which will significantly increase our US production capabilities.

PANDEMIC OVERVIEW

An influenza pandemic is a global epidemic that has the potential for severe morbidity and mortality.

Three influenza pandemics occurred during the 20th century: the 1918-1919 Spanish flu pandemic, the 1957 Asian flu pandemic and the 1968 Hong Kong flu pandemic. The Spanish flu pandemic was the most severe, causing over 500,000 deaths in the US and an estimated 20 to 40 million deaths worldwide.

The prospect of a pandemic is taking on increasing urgency because of the emergence of an H5N1 avian influenza strain in Southeast Asia 17 months ago. It continues to circulate and has the potential to mutate and become a human pandemic strain. To date, it has infected at least 97 people and killed more than half of its victims.[1] This is a completely new strain and epidemiologists believe the American population would be at risk if it spreads between humans.

Many experts believe that if this H5N1 virus sparks the next pandemic, it would most closely resemble the 1918 pandemic in terms of morbidity and mortality.[2]

According to the World Health Organization (WHO), the next pandemic is likely to result in 1 to 2.3 million hospitalizations and 280,000 to 650,000 deaths in industrialized nations alone. The US Centers for Disease Control and Prevention (CDC) estimated that as many as 207,000 Americans could die and up to 734,000 could be hospitalized during the next pandemic. Other estimates are even higher. Studies have estimated the costs of an influenza pandemic in the US between $71 billion and $166.5 billion. These estimates include only direct costs of medical care and indirect costs of lost productivity and mortality rates. Some experts have predicted that a major pandemic could bring the global economy to a halt.[3]

Sanofi pasteur recognizes the urgency of adequate preparation for a pandemic event and is taking steps to be ready.

---

[1] Remarks to the 58th World Health Assembly Plenary Session, Mike Leavitt. U.S. Department of Health and Human Services. Numbers updated on 5/23/05. Accessed May 17, 2005 at: http://www.hhs.gov/news/speech/2005/050516.html

[2] Osterholm MT. Preparing for the next pandemic. *N Engl J Med.* 2005 May 5;352(18):1839-42

[3] Osterholm MT. Preparing for the next pandemic. *N Engl J Med.* 2005 May 5;352(18):1839-42

PROGRESS TO DATE

We believe the expertise of vaccine manufacturers, particularly those with a track record in influenza vaccine production and distribution, should be utilized early in the planning process. Vaccines, by their very nature, are challenging to develop, produce and distribute. Manufacturers have a unique understanding of these challenges and can provide valuable process and policy input. Our knowledge and experience with the complexities of vaccine supply make industry an essential partner in pandemic planning and policy formulation.

The enormous public health threat posed by a potential pandemic prompted sanofi pasteur to re-examine our internal pandemic planning process. We have taken specific and deliberate steps toward a comprehensive pandemic strategy. We formed a global working group to examine preparedness, development, communications and legal issues. In the US, we have worked in cooperation with the US Department of Health and Human Services (HHS) to exchange ideas on how best to prepare for and respond to a pandemic influenza outbreak, and have provided significant input into the initial draft of its pandemic plan.

We have moved forward with clinical research and vaccine production because of important funding provided by Congress and the Administration. In May 2004, sanofi pasteur entered into the first of four pandemic agreements with the US government. The National Institute of Allergy and Infectious Diseases (NIAID) contracted with us to produce an investigational influenza vaccine based on the currently circulating H5N1 avian influenza virus strain. On March 10, 2005, in accordance with that agreement, sanofi pasteur delivered more than 8,000 investigational doses, which currently are being used in NIH-conducted clinical trials.

In September 2004, the company was awarded a second contract by HHS to produce two million bulk doses of an attenuated version of the same H5N1 avian influenza virus strain of vaccine. This contract represents an important step in gaining experience producing pandemic influenza vaccine on a large scale. This is critical because scale-up presents unique challenges in vaccine production. Part of our agreement is to determine the stability of this vaccine, which is important for understanding our ability to establish an H5N1 reserve.

Sanofi pasteur subsequently entered into a third agreement with HHS to establish and maintain flocks of egg-laying hens and to maintain other essential supplies. The goal is to ensure our ability to manufacture pandemic influenza vaccine at current full capacity levels on a year-round basis. Until now, egg availability has existed only on a seasonal basis to support normal influenza vaccine production. The agreement also calls for sanofi pasteur to manufacture, on an annual basis, investigational influenza vaccine of a candidate pandemic-like strain. Each year, HHS will identify the strain to be used in the investigational lot and will provide the reference virus on which each investigational lot will be based. This will enable us to gain experience working with various viral strains that might be similar to the next pandemic strain.

Finally, in April 2005, sanofi pasteur was awarded a fourth contract from HHS. This was to speed the development process for new cell culture influenza vaccines in the US and to design a US-based cell culture influenza vaccine manufacturing facility.

Required Action:

We are encouraged by the increased attention pandemic planning is receiving from the US government, industry, international agencies and key stakeholders. However, unresolved critical issues remain. The failure to address these challenges could adversely affect our country's ability to respond to a pandemic event.

I would like to briefly outline steps that should be taken to help the country better prepare for a pandemic and minimize the effects should one occur.

A first step is to steadily increase interpandemic influenza immunization rates. Manufacturers will respond to increased and predictable demand by producing additional vaccine to fulfill this demand.

This is important because our ability to produce and administer large quantities of influenza vaccine during interpandemic periods will enable a more rapid response during a pandemic. Increasing capacity in dedicated influenza vaccine production facilities and establishing an infrastructure that can deliver vaccine and immunize large numbers of people in a short period of time is a key component of pandemic preparedness.

To that end, Congress, industry and stakeholders need to work together to encourage higher influenza immunization rates in accordance with HHS' Healthy People 2010 immunization goals. The objective is to immunize approximately 180 million Americans. However, as a nation, we have never immunized more than 85 million people in any given year. This is unacceptable. A steady and sustained increase in interpandemic demand would give current manufacturers the confidence to continue expansion plans and new companies the incentive to enter the market.

Second, we need to ensure a proper combination of private and public sector distribution of vaccine in the event of a pandemic. We believe that while it will be important to establish mechanisms for mass immunizations and clinics, the private physicians' offices will continue to play a vital role as well. During a typical influenza season, the private sector distributes more than 85% of the nation's influenza supply. The private market provides maximum flexibility in vaccine distribution and allows us to reach large segments of the US population in their "medical homes." This includes the elderly, who should not stand in long lines and may be more comfortable with their personal physicians.

Last year's influenza vaccine shortage illustrated sanofi pasteur's unique expertise in processing and shipping product to virtually any location in the United States within 24-48 hours. We shipped vaccines to end-users in accordance with the CDC's recommendations and distribution plan. Further, the unprecedented degree of collaboration between sanofi pasteur and the CDC underscores our willingness to work with public agencies to protect America's public health. This year, sanofi pasteur has modified our ordering process to provide that, in the event of another shortage, available vaccine reaches high-risk people first. All of our "pre-book" customers are being asked to estimate what percentage of the vaccine they are requesting will be used for priority patients. The systems utilized to collect these data and the ability to easily identify priority recipients, as specified by federal, state and local governments, will be key in protecting the public health in the event of a pandemic. We also believe that there should be greater funding for coordinating communications between federal and state agencies and the private sector regarding vaccine allocation issues.

A third challenge is to continue to build pediatric stockpiles of all routinely recommended pediatric vaccines. When pandemic influenza strikes the United States, sanofi pasteur will have to slow down routine production, filling, and packaging for all other vaccines. We would have to shift personnel and other resources to optimize production and release of a monovalent pandemic influenza vaccine. Thus, it is essential that we resolve problems associated with the pediatric vaccine stockpile. HHS has appropriated funds but they have not been spent.

You may have read *The Washington Post* article on April 17, 2005 entitled "Pediatric Vaccine Stockpile at Risk." It pointed out that only 13 million of the requested 41 million doses of pediatric vaccine have been stockpiled due to a Securities and Exchange Commission rule that clarified standard accounting practices for a bill and hold sale. As a result, what had been a 20-year routine practice of stockpiling vaccines is no longer an option for sanofi pasteur. Over the last two years, we have been actively engaged in discussions with the CDC to address the issue. We encourage the Committee to help resolve the issues that surround the establishment of routine pediatric stockpiles in advance of a pandemic.

Pandemic influenza vaccine liability protection is another critical issue in pandemic preparedness. A special compensation and liability protection program will need to be established similar to the 1976 swine flu and 2002 smallpox model. Liability protection for companies is essential to ensure that manufacturers are able to fully participate in the development and licensure of a pandemic vaccine. This is of paramount importance. The new program should be completely distinct and separate from the existing Vaccine Injury Compensation Program (VICP). It should focus exclusively on liability protection for a monovalent influenza pandemic vaccine, precisely the type of vaccine that will be produced in a pandemic event. The failure to offer liability protection on a timely basis could have profound implications for the actual testing and development of large-scale production of vaccine, leaving the nation unprepared. It is important to address liability issues before a health emergency arises. This ensures that pandemic vaccines will be developed, economic costs will be mitigated, and the potential for needless and costly litigation will be curtailed.

We strongly urge Congress to consider—and establish—liability protections that are as strong as those afforded providers of smallpox vaccine under the Homeland Security Act of 2002. Vaccine liability provisions ensure that we can bring a pandemic influenza vaccine to market as quickly as possible.

Sanofi pasteur is committed to protecting America's public health in the fight against influenza through vaccinations. We want to commend Congress and the Administration for dedicating time and resources to this critical area. Thank you for giving us the opportunity to express our views on this important issue.

Mr. FERGUSON. Thank you very much. Dr. Iacuzio.

STATEMENT OF DOMINICK A. IACUZIO

Mr. IACUZIO. Mr. Chairman and the members of the sub-committee, I am Dr. Dominick Iacuzio, Medical Director for Tamiflu at Hoffmann-La Roche, a research-based pharmaceutical company. Prior to joining Roche, I worked at the NIH National Institute of Allergy and Infectious Diseases where I served as the Respiratory Diseases Branch Principal Technical Advisor for the Influenza Program. I am grateful for this opportunity to discuss the role of antiviral drugs and pandemic influenza preparedness and response, and I request that my full written testimony be submitted for the record.

As you have heard from the other witnesses today, pandemic influenza is one of our greatest public health threats. According to the Department of Homeland Security, a potential consequence for even a limited influenza pandemic could result in economic disruption, hospitalizations, and deaths far in excess of most terror attack scenarios.

Efforts to prepare for the pandemic threat cannot rely on vaccines alone. It is widely recognized that antiviral drug stockpiling is an important component of pandemic influenza preparedness. The Infectious Diseases Society of America has recommended, as you heard this morning, that the U.S. stockpile enough antiviral, up to 50 percent of the U.S. population.

Roche's Tamiflu is the leading prescription oral antiviral drug for influenza. Tamiflu was approved by the Food and Drug Administration in 1999 for treatment of Type A and B influenza and in 2000 for influenza prophylaxis or prevention. Fortunately, Tamiflu is well-tolerated with nausea and vomiting being most frequently reported as the adverse events. The efficacy of Tamiflu against Avian Influenza has been demonstrated by leading researchers and animal studies, in vitro data, and practical experience during the 2003 Avian Influenza outbreak in the Netherlands of H7N7. According to the World Health Organization, they have recommended use of Tamiflu to control the Avian Flu outbreaks in Asia.

Although the potential for resistance must be monitored carefully, no transmission of a Tamiflu-resistant virus in humans has been detected to date. It is imperative that Tamiflu be stockpiled in advance of a pandemic since inherent complexities in production severely limit our capability, our ability, to rapidly meet large-scale, unanticipated demand. The manufacturing process for Tamiflu takes 8 to 12 months from raw materials to finished product. The process involves many inputs and steps, including a unique starting material and a potentially explosive production step that can be carried out only in specialized and very costly facilities.

Historically, Roche has not produced the levels of Tamiflu required for global stockpiling. However, since 2003 we have increased total Tamiflu production capacity nearly eight-fold. Most importantly, early in our discussion HHS made several requests to Roche, all of which have been fulfilled. First, Roche has developed a U.S.-based supply chain. Second, Roche developed special U.S. packaging for stockpiled Tamiflu in order to extend dating and ease distribution and administration. Roche undertook these efforts in good faith and at great economic risk.

Roche is also developing a synthetic process for manufacturing the chemical used in the initial production step. This will ultimately reduce reliance on natural sources. Roche has received and is filing on schedule pandemic stockpile orders for Tamiflu from 25 countries worldwide. Discussions are underway for the U.S. Government to purchase significantly greater amounts of Tamiflu. However, HHS stockpile purchases to date are sufficient to treat less than 1 percent of the U.S. population. We have also received a non-bonding letter of intent for HHS to purchase additional treatments to cover under 2 percent of the population.

In contrast, countries such as the United Kingdom, France, Finland, Norway, Switzerland, and New Zealand are ordering enough Tamiflu to cover between 20 and 40 percent of their populations. Unfortunately, given the complexities I have described, the increasing global demand, any government that does not stockpile sufficient quantities of Tamiflu in advance cannot be assured of an adequate supply at the outbreak of an influenza pandemic.

If I can leave you with three messages from my testimony today, they are the following: first, there is a consensus by global health authorities that Tamiflu is effective and an important tool in pandemic influenza preparedness and response; second, that other nations are currently well ahead of the United States in Tamiflu stockpiling; and finally, the U.S. has to make commitment now to ensure a timely and adequate supply of Tamiflu. We at Roche want to continue to work closely with the subcommittee and HHS to assist the U.S. in ensuring pandemic preparedness. On behalf of Roche, thank you for highlighting this critical issue, and I will be pleased to answer any questions that you may have.

[The prepared statement of Dominick A. Iacuzio follows:]

PREPARED STATEMENT OF DOMINICK A. IACUZIO, MEDICAL DIRECTOR, HOFFMANN-LA ROCHE INC.

Mr. Chairman and Members of the Subcommittee, I am Dr. Dominick Iacuzio, Medical Director at Hoffmann-La Roche Inc. ("che"), a research-based pharmaceutical company. Since joining Roche, I have been the medical officer responsible for Tamiflu® (oseltamivir phosphate), the world's first oral medication effective against the type A and B strains of the influenza virus. Prior to joining Roche, I worked at the National Institute of Allergy and Infectious Diseases, National Institutes of Health, where I served as the Respiratory Disease Branch's principal technical advisor for the Influenza Program. I am grateful for this opportunity to discuss with you the role of antiviral drugs in pandemic influenza preparedness and response, and I commend the Subcommittee for its efforts to protect the American people against this very real public health threat.

THE PANDEMIC INFLUENZA THREAT

Every year, seasonal influenza causes an average of 36,000 deaths and 114,000 hospitalizations.[1] In addition to the annual influenza seasons, three influenza pandemics took place during the 20th century. In 1918, approximately 500,000 people died from the so-called "Spanish Flu," and up to 50 million may have died worldwide. The 1957-58 "Asian flu" killed 70,000 Americans, and the 1968-69 "Hong Kong flu" caused over 34,000 deaths in this country.[2] An influenza pandemic occurs when an existing influenza strain mutates. The emergence of such a new viral strain, the lack of previous exposure and immunity to the virus, and the lack of a vaccine that can protect against the new strain can

---

[1] Department of Health and Human Services, *Draft Pandemic Influenza Response and Preparedness Plan, Core Document,* 14 (Aug. 2004), *available at* http://www.hhs.gov/nvpo/pandemicplan/finalpandemiccore.pdf.

[2] Centers for Disease Control and Prevention, *Fact Sheet: Information About Influenza Pandemics* (March 8, 2005).

72

ignite a global influenza epidemic, i.e., a pandemic. It has been 36 years since the last influenza pandemic, thanks in large part to the development of influenza vaccinations, as well as methods to predict influenza strains and redesign vaccines annually to include the strains predicted to affect the population in a given year.

However, it appears that the factors associated with a pandemic are now moving into place. First, we have a highly pathogenic strain of avian influenza circulating widely in Asia. Second, this avian strain appears to be increasingly capable of causing deadly disease in humans and animals. In fact, the avian virus has been fatal in approximately 60 percent of people infected by it.[3] While efficient human-to-human transmission of the virus—the final barrier to an influenza pandemic—has yet to occur, it is possible—if not probable—that persons harboring both human and avian influenza viruses could become "mixing vessels" from which a new virus emerges that is easily transmitted among humans. Indeed, a recent World Health Organization (WHO) assessment noted that new epidemiological findings in Asia indicate that the virus may be becoming more capable of human-to-human transmission.[4]

Make no mistake: should an influenza pandemic occur, the threat to the U.S. public would be great. In its draft *Pandemic Influenza Preparedness and Response Plan* (Plan), the U.S. Department of Health and Human Services (HHS) recognizes an influenza pandemic as having "a greater potential to cause rapid increases in death and illness than virtually any other natural health threat.[5] Health experts estimate that if the virus is passed efficiently between humans, avian flu could result in a pandemic causing over 50 million deaths worldwide.[6] Studies cited recently by the Centers for Disease Control and Prevention (CDC) estimate that, without vaccines or drugs, a "medium level" pandemic would kill between 89,000 and 207,000 Americans, and sicken another 20 to 47 million—causing up to 42 million outpatient visits and 734,000 hospitalizations.[7] In fact, according to the Department of Homeland Security, the potential consequences of even a limited influenza pandemic could result in deaths, hospitalizations and economic disruption far in excess of most terror attack scenarios.[8] In addition to the human toll, the economic cost of such a pandemic has been estimated at $71 to $167 billion.[9] Without a doubt, planning for such a global health crisis must be a major public health priority.

Both the HHS Plan and the WHO *Global Influenza Preparedness Plan* emphasize that adequately addressing the threat of a pandemic influenza outbreak will require availability of both an influenza vaccine and antiviral drugs.[10] If available, vaccines, which typically are administered before an outbreak of influenza, can provide an effective defense against developing seasonal or pandemic influenza, as well as in slowing transmission among humans.

However, vaccines have important limitations. First, accurately predicting the specific viral strain or strains that ultimately may cause an influenza pandemic cannot be assured. Consequently, effective vaccines may not be available at the time a pandemic outbreak is first detected. Second, the propensity of viruses to mutate can lead to the rapid generation of new strains. Thus, there is a possibility that a vaccine effective against the viral strain accountable for the outbreak may be impotent against the virus' mutated progeny. This is one reason why unique vaccines to guard against seasonal influenza must be produced, licensed, and distributed each year, and thus, cannot be stockpiled for use against multiple outbreaks. Finally, given the pace of an outbreak of pandemic influenza, initial reliance on vaccines may not be feasible. For example, the WHO estimates it will take six to nine

---

[3] World Health Organization, *Cumulative Number of Confirmed Human Cases of Avian Influenza A/(H5N1) Reported to WHO* (May 19, 2005), *available at* http://www.who.int/csr/disease/avian_influenza/country/cases_table_2005_05_19/en/print.html.

[4] World Health Organization, *Inter-country Consultation, Influenza A/H5N1 in Humans in Asia* (May 6-7, 2005).

[5] Department of Health and Human Services, *Draft Pandemic Influenza Response and Preparedness Plan, Executive Summary* 3, (Aug. 2004), *available at* http://www.hhs.gov/nvpo/pandemicplan.

[6] World Health Organization, *Estimating the Impact of the Next Influenza Pandemic: Enhancing Preparedness* (Dec. 8, 2004), *available at* http://www.who.int/csr/disease/influenza/preparedness2004_12_08/en/index.html.

[7] Centers for Disease Control and Prevention, *Influenza Pandemic Fact Sheet* (Mar. 8, 2005), *available at* http://www.cdc.gov/flu/avian/gen-info/pandemics.htm.

[8] *15 Nightmares for Disaster Planning*, N.Y. Times (March 16, 2005).

[9] CDC, *Influenza Pandemic Fact Sheet*.

[10] Department of Health and Human Services, *Draft Pandemic Influenza Response and Preparedness Plan, Core Document* 23 (Aug. 2004), available at http://www.hhs.gov/nvpo/pandemicplan/finalpandemiccore.pdf; World Health Organization, *WHO Global Influenza Preparedness Plan* 13 (2005), *available at* http://www.who.int/csr/resources/publications/influenza/WHO_CDS_CSR_GIP_2005_5.pdf.

months to develop a vaccine effective against the circulating pandemic virus strain.[11] Of course, producing and distributing the vaccine on a large scale also will take considerable time, and a vaccine, once administered, may take several weeks to trigger immunity, or require multiple administrations.

For all of these reasons, HHS and the WHO have recommended that efforts to prepare for an influenza pandemic not rely on vaccines alone. As stated in a recent WHO report, "[p]ending the availability of vaccines, antiviral agents will be the principal medical intervention for reducing morbidity and mortality, which becomes the most important priority once a pandemic is underway.[12] Notably, certain antiviral drugs can be used either to treat the flu or as a prophylactic to prevent those at risk from becoming infected. Recently published models suggest that an influenza pandemic could be contained if 80 percent of those exposed to the virus used targeted antiviral drugs prophylactically.[13]

Finally, antivirals have four additional characteristics that warrant their inclusion in any influenza pandemic plan: (1) antivirals have a long shelf-life, permitting them to be stockpiled for several years, and thus immediately available when an outbreak occurs; (2) antiviral drugs begin to work immediately after they are administered; (3) certain antivirals work against multiple types of influenza; and (4) utilization of antivirals does not interfere with immunologic response.

THE ROLE OF TAMIFLU ® IN AN INFLUENZA PANDEMIC

Roche's Tamiflu ® (oseltamivir phosphate) is the leading prescription oral antiviral drug. Tamiflu ® was approved by the Food and Drug Administration (FDA) in 1999 for the treatment of type A and B influenza. Specifically, Tamiflu ®, a neuraminidase inhibitor, works by attacking the influenza virus and its ability to replicate, rather than simply addressing influenza symptoms. Tamiflu ® is indicated for treatment of patients one year and older, and, if taken within forty-eight hours of the onset of symptoms, can help patients recover from the flu faster. As a prophylactic, an indication approved in 2000, Tamiflu ® is labeled for use by adults and adolescents 13 years of age and older, although data on children one year of age and older have recently been submitted to FDA for review. Tamiflu ® has a low likelihood of clinically significant drug interactions and is generally well-tolerated, with nausea and vomiting being the most frequently reported adverse events. Tamiflu ® is available in both capsule and pediatric suspension form.

As CDC Director Dr. Julie Gerberding informed this Subcommittee in a November 2004 hearing, Tamiflu ® "is the only antiviral drug known to be effective against avian influenza.[14] The efficacy of Tamiflu ® against avian influenza has been demonstrated in animal studies by leading researchers, *in vitro* data, and practical experience during an avian influenza outbreak in the Netherlands.[15] Accordingly, the WHO has recommended use of Tamiflu ® in those potentially exposed to avian flu in Asia.[16] Additionally, while a possibility exists for an influenza virus to emerge with decreased sensitivity to any antiviral drug, the Tamiflu ®-resistant viruses isolated in humans to date do not appear to be effectively transmissible.[17]

---

[11] World Health Organization (WHO) Global Influenza Preparedness Plan: The Role of WHO and Recommendations for National Measures Before and During Pandemics (Apr. 2005), *available at* http://www.who.int/ csr/resources/publications/influenza/WHO_CDS_CSR_EDC_99_1/en/print.html.

[12] World Health Organization, *Avian Influenza: Assessing the Pandemic Threat* (Jan. 2005), *available at* http://www.who.int/csr/disease/influenza/H5N1-9reduit.pdf.

[13] N.M. Ferguson et al., *A Population-Dynamic Model for Evaluating the Potential Spread of Drug-Resistant Influenza Virus Infections During Community-Based Use of Antivirals,* 51 Journal of Antimicrobial Chemotherapy 977 (2003); I.M. Longini et al., *Containing Pandemic Influenza with Antiviral Agents,* 159 Am. J. Epidemiology 623 (2004).

[14] *Flu Vaccine and Protecting High-Risk Individuals: Hearing Before the Subcomm. on Health of the House Comm. on Energy & Commerce* 108th Cong. (Nov. 18, 2004) (Statement of Dr. Julie Gerberding).

[15] I.A. Leneva et al., *The Neuraminidase Inhibitor GS4104 (Oseltamivir Phosphate) is Efficacious Against A/Hong Kong/156/97 (H5N1) and A/Hong Kong/1074/99 (H9N2) Influenza Viruses,* 48 Antiviral Res 101 (2000).

[16] World Health Organization, *WHO Interim Guidelines for Health Monitoring of Persons Involved in Culling of Animals Potentially Infected with Highly Pathogenic Avian Influenza Viruses* (Mar. 22, 2004), available at http://www.wpro.who.int/avian_flu/docs/Health_monitor_person.asp.

[17] Data collected from patients treated with Tamiflu ®, at its approved dose and for the approved treatment duration, demonstrate an overall incidence of resistant virus of only 0.4 percent in adults and four percent in children aged one to 12. All of the resistant virus strains were found unlikely to spread within a community, even under conditions of widespread Tamiflu ® use for both treatment and prevention of influenza. N. Roberts, *Treatment of Influenza*

Continued

For the prevention of influenza in those 13 years or older, Tamiflu® is administered following close contact with an infected individual who demonstrates characteristic symptoms of influenza, and based on knowledge that influenza is circulating in the area for 10 days, or up to six weeks for seasonal prophylaxis. The approved dose and duration of treatment—75mg twice daily for five days—is expected to represent the minimum required for the management of an influenza pandemic. To ensure Tamiflu® remains effective against the influenza virus, Roche does not recommend strategies which may utilize lower doses or shorter duration of therapy compared with the recommended dose.

ALTHOUGH ROCHE IS TAKING STEPS TO INCREASE TAMIFLU® PRODUCTION, THE U.S. GOVERNMENT MUST MAKE CONTRACTUAL STOCKPILE COMMITMENTS TO ENSURE A ROBUST U.S. ANTIVIRAL DRUG SUPPLY

As noted, both HHS and the WHO include stockpiling of antiviral drugs as a central component of their developing plans for influenza pandemic preparedness. Both the Infectious Diseases Society of America (IDSA) and the WHO have recently acknowledged that Tamiflu®, in particular, is uniquely suited to pandemic stockpiling, for several reasons: (1) its efficacy against influenza types A and B; (2) the absence of a known Tamiflu®-resistant virus transmissible in humans; and (3) the product's five-year shelf life.

It is imperative that Tamiflu® be stockpiled in advance of the outbreak of a pandemic because inherent complexities in production severely limit capacity to rapidly meet large-scale, unanticipated demand. The manufacturing process for Tamiflu® is complex, and takes 8-12 months from raw materials to finished product. The process involves many intermediate steps, including a unique starting material, and a potentially explosive production step that can be carried out only in specialized and costly facilities. Given these complexities, significant lead time is needed to increase production capacity and build stockpiles of the quantity required for an influenza pandemic.

Historically, Roche has produced enough Tamiflu® to meet the seasonal influenza demand. For example, just over one million prescriptions for Tamiflu® were written in 2003 in the United States, while preceding years averaged 600,000 to 700,000 prescriptions. In contrast, the IDSA has recommended that the government stockpile enough antiviral drugs to treat up to 50 percent of the U.S. population.[18]

Despite the obstacles I have described, the company doubled production capacity at our European facility from 2003 to 2004, and we are doing so again during 2005. Roche plans additional expansion of production capacity for Tamiflu® in 2006. Most importantly, early in our discussions HHS made several requests to Roche, all of which we have fulfilled. First, Roche has developed a U.S.-based supply chain. When that supply chain is launched later this year, total Tamiflu® active pharmaceutical ingredient and capsule production capacity will have increased globally by nearly eight-fold over production capacity in 2003. Second, Roche developed special U.S. packaging for stockpiled Tamiflu in order to extend dating and ease distribution and administration. Roche undertook these efforts in good faith and at great economic risk. Moreover, Roche is developing a synthetic process for manufacturing the chemical used in the initial production step, which will ultimately reduce reliance on natural sources.

Roche has received and is filling—on schedule—pandemic stockpile orders for Tamiflu® from 25 countries worldwide. Discussions are underway for the U.S. government to purchase for its stockpile significantly greater amounts of Tamiflu® for this year and beyond. However, HHS stockpile purchases to date total approximately 2.3 million courses of treatment, or enough to treat less than one percent of the U.S. population. We have also received a non-binding letter of intent for HHS to purchase an additional three million courses of treatment, or enough to cover under two percent of the population. In contrast, countries such as the United Kingdom, France, Finland, Norway, Switzerland and New Zealand are ordering enough Tamiflu® to cover between 20 to 40 percent of their populations.

---

with Neuraminidase Inhibitors: Virological Implications, 356 Philosophical Transactions of the Royal Society 1895 (2001).

[18] World Health Organization, *Governments in a Dilemma Over Bird Flu: Uncertainty Over the Risk Posed by Bird Flu to Human Health Has Left Policymakers in a Dilemma* (May 1, 2005), *available at* http://www.who.int/bulletin/volumes/83/5/infocus0505/en/index1.html; Infectious Diseases Society of America *IDSA's Principles For Action Needed to Prepare the U.S. to Effectively Respond to Interpandemic/Pandemic Influenza* (Mar. 10, 2005), *available at* http://www.idsociety.org/Template.cfm?Section=Search & CONTENTID=10445&TEMPLATE=/Content Management/ContentDisplay.cfm.

Unfortunately, given the complexities I have described, any government that does not stockpile sufficient quantities of Tamiflu® in advance cannot be assured an adequate supply at the outbreak of an influenza pandemic. We are greatly concerned that with the continually increasing global demand for Tamiflu®, and in the absence of a long-term U.S. commitment to stockpile the product, U.S.-manufactured Tamiflu® may have to be exported to countries with committed orders. While Roche commends HHS for its efforts to date, we cannot emphasize enough the immediate need for the United States government to make the contractual commitments necessary to ensure that an adequate stockpile is developed to meet the looming pandemic threat.

Alerted to the pandemic threat, governments now have an unprecedented opportunity to attempt to minimize the catastrophic loss of life, debilitating illness, and enormous economic costs that a pandemic could wreak on the United States and the world. If I can leave you with three messages from my testimony today, they are the following. First, there is a consensus by leading global health authorities that Tamiflu® is effective and an important tool in pandemic preparedness and response. Second, other nations are currently well ahead of the United States in Tamiflu® stockpiling. Finally, there are important practical constraints on the production of Tamiflu® that make immediate U.S. contractual commitments for future pandemic supplies a necessity.

We at Roche want to continue to work closely with this Subcommittee, HHS, and governments around the world to assist in ensuring our pandemic preparedness. On behalf of Roche, thank you for highlighting the importance of this critical issue, and I will be pleased to answer any questions you may have.

Mr. FERGUSON. Thank you very much. Dr. Tripp.

STATEMENT OF RALPH A. TRIPP

Mr. TRIPP. Mr. Chairman and members of the subcommittee, I am here today to tell you about the emerging pandemic threat of Avian Influenza and how scientists at the University of Georgia in collaboration with Alnylam Pharmaceuticals in Cambridge, Massachusetts are developing novel and proven therapeutics to prevent Avian Influenza virus and other important respiratory virus infections. My comments today echo those concerns of the CDC, World Health Organization, and Institute of Medicine, and others about the need for preparing for pandemic flu.

I am keenly aware of the threat that mankind faces by influenza and other important respiratory viruses having worked at the Center for Disease Control for 7 years in the Respiratory and Enteric Viruses Branch before moving to the University of Georgia to become the Georgia Research Alliance Eminent Scholar in vaccine development, as well as the director of the Center for Disease Intervention there. And I must reemphasize the imminent threat of an influenza pandemic.

As we are all aware, pandemic flu spreads rapidly and during the pandemics of 1957 and 1968, those viruses took less than 3 to 4 months to go from the site of origin in Southeast Asia to North America and Europe. Clearly, the conditions are more favorable for spread these days with the air travel possibilities so an outbreak could occur in a matter of days around cities throughout the world. Once a pandemic flu emerges, we probably won't be able to prevent the global spread, but if we are prepared with things such as antivirals, it can significantly reduce its impact.

The current outbreak of flu in Asia known as H5N1 is thought to have significantly heightened the risk of another flu pandemic as reported by the World Health Organization. Since the emergence of H5N1 in poultry in mid-December 2003, this strain has devastated the poultry industry in nine different countries in

Southeast Asia. Clearly, it would have a similar impact if it came to the United States.

There has also been numerous reports of human infection by this strain, as has been described by the witnesses today. Scientists at the University in Georgia, in collaboration with investigators at the Center for Disease Control and Alnylam Pharmaceuticals, recognize that multiple approaches are going to be necessary to protect the human population from the newly emerging virus strains such as H5N1.

Vaccines are obviously the mainstay of prophylaxis against influenza, but there are technical and safety issues that we have all heard about that must be overcome. These include difficulty in predicting which strains of virus may emerge, difficulty in preparing sufficient quantities of the vaccine to meet the global demand, and clearly in storage and distribution of these vaccines.

Antivirals have been shown to be very effective in treating common influenza. However, as you have heard, H5N1, Avian Flu is resistant to two of the most common drugs, rimantadine and amantadine and now they is some evidence and literature that the virus may be developing resistance to a newly developed drug Tamiflu or oseltamivir. The evidence for viral resistance to antiviral drugs indicates that more than one drug is going to be necessary to combat emerging flu and new, novel approaches are going to be necessary to enhance effectiveness of these drugs, as well as to prevent viral resistance to the existing drugs.

In my laboratory at the University of Georgia we are working with new, breakthrough technology with Alnylam Pharmaceuticals called RNA interference. RNA interference is a natural process. It occurs in all the cells of our body. The process is meted by activity of short strands of RNA that silence host genes and control development. We have been able to harness that power to actually generally RNA-interfering drugs that prevent respiratory virus infection, particularly for respiratory syncytial virus. And now we have shown that with these same RNA interference drugs are useful in preventing infection by highly pathogenic H5N1 and H7 strains of flu.

We have also shown these RNA interference drugs are useful both prophylactically and therapeutically to prevent respiratory syncytial virus, and this is a virus that is the leading cause of series lower respiratory tract illness in infants and young children worldwide for which there is no vaccine and treatments are limited.

So the studies from my laboratory at the University of Georgia have shown the potential to create powerful therapeutics that meet the demand for new drugs with higher potency, lower toxicity, and having a much higher degree of specificity in that they only attack the cells that are affected by the virus.

So given the pending threat of influenza, it is absolutely necessary that our disease intervention strategies move beyond the standard vaccine and into a new class of proven preventative and therapeutic treatments. With RNA interference, the creation of a safer and more accurate antiviral is certainly within reach and on the horizon. These specific antiviral therapeutics can be developed rapidly, they can produce the high levels, and they can be stockpiled or stored as needed.

So I am here today to urge the Members of Congress to bring universities like the University of Georgia together with private sector companies like Alnylam Pharmaceuticals to develop breakthrough solutions to address the important human diseases like pandemic flu and provide alternatives to antiviral drugs, certainly which some have become resistant to.

Support for this new and proven technology will provide an unprecedented means to control pandemic flu, as well as address other important viral infections. And clearly, without support for this type of a robust research program, we are destined to relive the pandemics of the past. And in developing these RNA-interfering drugs, we are developing new tools to address any emerging infectious virus. And I would like to thank you for your time.

[The prepared statement of Ralph A. Tripp follows:]

PREPARED STATEMENT OF RALPH A. TRIPP, DIRECTOR, CENTER FOR DISEASE INTERVENTION

SUMMARY

The World Health Organization (WHO) and influenza experts worldwide warn that an influenza virus (flu) pandemic is inevitable and imminent and will likely be caused by widespread distribution of an avian influenza virus, e.g. avian flu.

Vaccines are the mainstay of prophylaxis against influenza, but there is currently no vaccine capable of protecting humans from infection with avian flu.Currently approved anti-viral drugs may be useful to treat pandemic flu but their effectiveness is limited by development of resistance.

Novel and new anti-viral approaches are required to enhance the effectiveness of existing anti-viral drugs, prevent viral resistance to existing drugs, and to provide a strategy to combat avian flu and other important respiratory viral diseases.

The discovery of *RNA interference, or RNAi* has revolutionized our ability to offer new, potent and specific viral disease intervention. RNAi is a natural biological process that occurs in all of our cells. The process is mediated by the activity of short strands of RNA that specifically silence the targeted gene of interest.

We have harnessed the power of RNAi to silence respiratory virus infection and disease by targeting viral genes. We have shown that RNAi is very potent, specific, and reactive for all strains of virus targeted.

RNAi is a new breakthrough solution to address pandemic flu that is on the horizon. Support for this new and proven technology will provide an unprecedented means to control pandemic flu and other important respiratory virus infections that carry a high disease burden on mankind.

Pandemic Influenza (flu):

A pandemic is an epidemic that spreads rapidly around the world with high rates of illness and death. While people are exposed to different strains of the flu virus many times in their lives, about three or four times every century a radically different strain of flu causes a pandemic.

Such warnings by the World Health Organization, Centers for Disease Control, National Institutes of Health and Institute of Medice have been fueled by the persistence of a highly virulent strain of avian influenza virus in Asia that experts fear could trigger another influenza pandemic.

Influenza pandemics are not new. In the 20th century, mankind has faced three influenza pandemics. The first was the devastating 1918 "Spanish Flu" pandemic, as well as two less severe influenza pandemics in 1957 and 1968.

Key facts of pandemic flu:

Pandemic flu occurs every few decades and spreads rapidly to affect most countries and regions around the world. Unlike the "ordinary" flu that usually occurs every winter, pandemic flu can occur at any time of year

Pandemic flu is much more serious than "ordinary" flu—as much as a quarter of the population may be affected—maybe more.

A serious pandemic is also likely to cause many deaths, disrupt the daily life of many people and cause intense pressure on health, poultry and other industries.

What is pandemic flu caused by?

The emergence of a new flu virus which is markedly different from recently circulating strains and to which few people have any immunity.

Strategies to protect against pandemic flu:

Vaccines are the mainstay of prophylaxis against influenza, but there are technical and safety issues that must be overcome, and problems in producing sufficient vaccine to meet global requirements. There is no vaccine ready to protect against pandemic flu.

Currently approved anti-viral drugs can be used to treat pandemic flu but their effectiveness is limited by development of drug resistance.

The nature of the next pandemic flu: Avian Influenza:

WHO and influenza experts worldwide are concerned that the recent appearance and widespread distribution of an avian influenza virus, influenza A/H5N1 (H5N1) "has the potential to ignite the next pandemic", World Health Organization, December 2004.

What is Avian Influenza?

Avian influenza is a contagious disease of birds and poultry caused by influenza A viruses. All bird species are susceptible to infection, but domestic poultry flocks are especially vulnerable. Infection can cause epidemics associated with severe illness, high death rates, and economic devastation.

Where does Avian Influenza occur?

Avian flu occurs worldwide. The current outbreak of highly pathogenic avian flu (H5N1) began in Asia and has to date affected poultry in nine countries in Asia. In three of these countries, H5N1 strain has also infected people.

How does Avian Influenza spread?

Avian flu is spread in poultry flocks either via respiratory secretions or contact with contaminated droppings. People are usually infected through close contact with infected birds or their feces. Person-to-person spread, so far appears to difficult.

Protecting the human population from Avian Influenza:

There is currently no vaccine capable of protecting humans from infection, and effectiveness of existing anti-virals is not well understood.

Why I am here today:

I am here today to tell you about the emerging pandemic threat from avian influenza virus and how scientists at the University of Georgia are developing novel therapeutics with Alnylam Pharmaceuticals, Cambridge, MA to treat and prevent avian influenza and other important respiratory viral infections.

My concerns echo those of the Centers for Disease Control, National Institutes of Health, the World Health Organization, and Institute of Medicine which all warn of the need for pandemic flu preparedness, particularly for avian influenza.

What is the potential impact of Avian Influenza?

The emergence of new influenza A virus subtypes have caused all three known flu pandemics, all of which spread around the world within 1 year of being detected.

1918-19, "Spanish flu", [H1N1]: caused the highest number of known influenza deaths: more than 500,000 people died in the United States, and up to 50 million people may have died worldwide. Nearly half of those who died were young, healthy adults. Influenza A (H1N1) viruses still circulate today after being introduced again into the human population in the 1970s.

1957-58, "Asian flu," [H2N2], caused about 70,000 deaths in the United States. First identified in China in late February 1957, the Asian flu spread to the United States by June 1957.

1968-69, "Hong Kong flu," [H3N2), caused about 34,000 deaths in the United States. This virus was first detected in Hong Kong in early 1968 and spread to the United States later that year. Influenza A (H3N2) viruses still circulate today.

Historical patterns and influenza:

Influenza pandemics can be expected to occur, on average, three to four times each century when new virus subtypes emerge and are readily transmitted from person-to-person.

Pandemic flu spreads rapidly. During the pandemics of 1957 and 1968, the viruses took only 3-4 months to spread from southeast Asia—where they were first identified—to Europe and North America.

Today, conditions are far more favorable to the spread flu. With high population density, and ease of air travel around the world, an outbreak could spread to virtually every city in the world in a matter of a few days.

Influenza virus disease intervention strategies:

Multiple approaches will be required to protect the human population from newly emerging influenza virus strains such as H5N1 and others.

Vaccines are the mainstay of prophylaxis against influenza, but there are technical and safety issues that must be overcome.

Anti-viral agents have been shown to be effective toward treating influenza subtypes; however, avian flu (H5N1) is resistant to two common influenza drugs, rimantadine and amantadine, but newly developed drugs such as Tamiflu and Relenza appear to be somewhat effective.

The evidence for viral resistance to anti-viral agents indicates that more than one drug will be necessary to combat influenza.

Novel new anti-viral approaches—RNA Interference (RNAi):

New anti-viral drugs are required to enhance the effectiveness of current drugs and prevent drug resistance.

In my laboratory at the University of Georgia, we are working with new breakthrough technology called RNA interference, or RNAi. RNAi is a natural biological process that occurs in all of our cells to control development. RNAi is mediated by the activity of short strands of RNA that specifically silence the targeted gene of interest.

We have harnessed the power of RNAi to silence respiratory virus infection and disease by targeting viral genes. We have shown that RNAi is very potent, specific, and reactive for all strains of virus targeted. We have shown that RNAi prophylaxis and therapeutic treatment can be used to effectively silence respiratory syncytial virus (RSV) which is the leading cause of serious lower respiratory tract in infants and young children worldwide.

RNAi has the potential to create powerful therapeutics that meet the demand for new drugs with higher potency, lower toxicity, and have a high degree of specificity, i.e. only attack their target and do so very efficiently.

RNAi and the pending threat of pandemic flu:

It is absolutely necessary that our disease intervention strategies move beyond the standard vaccine and into a new class of proven preventative and therapeutic treatments. With RNAi, the creation of a safer, more accurate and efficient anti-viral treatment for pandemic influenza is closer in reach.

Specific anti-viral RNAi therapeutics can be developed rapidly, i.e. within several months, produced at high levels, and stock piled or stored as needed.

RNAi is a new breakthrough solution to address pandemic flu that is on the horizon. Support for this new and proven technology will provide an unprecedented means to control pandemic flu and other important respiratory virus infections that carry a high disease burden on mankind.

Clearly, without support for this robust research program that can prevent respiratory virus disease burden, and silence virus replication and spread, we are doomed to relive the pandemics of the past. In developing the RNAi disease intervention strategies, we are developing tools to respond to any novel virus that may emerge.

Mr. FERGUSON. Thank you very much to all of you, and with that we will begin some questioning. The Chair recognizes himself for the purpose of some questions.

Dr. Iacuzio, Dr. Gerberding in the testimony in the first panel talked about Tamiflu when I was asking her questions about antivirals, which seemed to be at odds with some testimony that she had given last November. And I know that, Dr. Pavia, you said you had some disagreements with some things that Dr. Gerberding said earlier today. Specifically about the effectiveness of Tamiflu with some strains of the Avian Flu, Dr. Tripp just referenced that as well. How does what Dr. Gerberding was saying square with your knowledge—I mean, you make it—how does that square with your understanding of the effectiveness of Tamiflu with regard to various strains of the Avian Flu?

Mr. IACUZIO. There is scientifically published literature that oseltamivir, Tamiflu, has been tested in the lab against all known subtypes of Type A influenza, including all Avian strains, N1 through the N9, which basically—you know, they cover all the Type A viruses, and it is effective against all those in the laboratory.

In addition, we have talked with officials, Klaus Stohr at the World Health Organization about the latest data that he is aware of from the Asian outbreak of Avian Flu out there, and according to the notes that I have is that no deaths from any individuals who have taken Tamiflu within the first 48 hours have been reported to his knowledge. So this is what the WHO is aware of as of this point in time.

Mr. FERGUSON. I just want to make sure that there isn't some new data, new information since last November when Dr. Gerberding testified in front of Congress. She said she believed Tamiflu was highly effective for strains that were known. Is there anything new in the last several months that would challenge that notion?

Mr. IACUZIO. No, there really isn't. There had been reports of increased resistance reported in one paper in Japan, but the data was from a study where children are one, underdosed; two, they are not given the dose at the long enough duration; and three, the isolates were isolated through a highly sophisticated laboratory technology, which we don't know what that means. I mean they were basically laboratory curiosities. We don't believe that these are infectious strains.

Mr. FERGUSON. So given that the data that you have and published studies that you cited——

Mr. IACUZIO. Right.

Mr. FERGUSON. [continuing] there seems to be a consensus that Tamiflu is effective for Avian Flu, yet we have heard from GAO and others that it seems to be inadequate, I guess, to put it mildly. Our efforts to stockpile antivirals to prepare for this—what everyone seems to think is an eventuality—seems to be not the most aggressive course of action that we could be taking. You have been in discussions—Roche has been in discussions with the U.S. Government for 2 years or so to negotiate the production of more Tamiflu for stockpiling purposes. Obviously, negotiations that take 2 years or more, every day that is lost is precious time when additional antivirals could be being produced and stockpiled. Given that, we are where we are.

If an order were placed tomorrow—we have heard World Health Organization and others have recommended 25 to 50 percent of the population should have the ability to be covered. You mentioned a number of countries which have already placed orders or have begun stockpiling orders to cover 20 to 40 percent of their population. If the United States placed an order for Tamiflu tomorrow to cover 25 percent of our population, perhaps on the conservative side of what many of these other countries are doing, what would be the timeline for production? How would that affect your production capacity? What would be the timeline for your ability to produce that? And is there any way, if that is not real fast, that you would be able to make investments or to be able to streamline that or advance that timeline any quicker?

Mr. IACUZIO. Since we began the conversations with public health officials in 2003, Roche globally has increased production capability eight-fold. Since locally we were—a year ago, February 2004 we were requested for considering a U.S. production facility. Roche has, as I said in my statement, has taken that initiative and that production facility we expect to up and running by the third quarter of 2005, this year. With that increased capacity both globally and the U.S. we would be able to produce—because of existing orders that already have been booked—about three million doses this fiscal year, by the end of this year; 13 million doses that are remaining for 2006; and by the end of 2007, another additional 70 million doses. So by the end of 2007 we should be able to provide approximately enough for 25 percent of the U.S. population.

Mr. FERGUSON. That is your capacity? That is what you would be able to do?

Mr. IACUZIO. If orders came in now because every day that goes by additional countries are placing orders——

Mr. FERGUSON. What has been ordered—what has the United States ordered thus far?

Mr. IACUZIO. Right now we have firm commitment—well, the U.S. has purchased 2.3 million doses, and there is a non-binding letter of agreement for an additional, I believe, three million doses.

Mr. FERGUSON. So we are talking about less than six million doses——

Mr. IACUZIO. Right.

Mr. FERGUSON. [continuing] that the U.S. would be stockpiling?

Mr. IACUZIO. At this point in time.

Mr. FERGUSON. Is that enough?

Mr. IACUZIO. I think that is a question really for public health officials.

Mr. FERGUSON. Dr. Pavia, is that enough?

Mr. PAVIA. It is clearly not enough. I think to find the right number using good epidemiologic techniques is something we haven't done yet——

Mr. FERGUSON. Yes, but we can all agree that——

Mr. PAVIA. [continuing] but the current amount——

Mr. FERGUSON. [continuing] this is imperfect—estimating what we would need is an imperfect science, but I think something that we could probably all agree on is that six million doses doesn't come close to being able to prepare us for what we all agree is the eventuality of this catastrophe.

Mr. PAVIA. It is a painfully small amount to have to use.

Mr. FERGUSON. I am over my time. Mr. Allen.

Mr. ALLEN. Thank you. Thank you, Mr. Chairman. And I want to thank all members of the panel.

Mr. Hosbach, I wanted to ask you about what incentives industry needs to increase production capacity in the U.S. but I think you pretty much answered that. I mean you said increase vaccination rates for annual flus, get a public and private distribution system in place, do vaccine liability protection, and four, CDC would have to build the capacity to increase stockpiles. Is there anything you would add to those four? Is there anything you want to elaborate on that? Because, you know, how do we get—obviously there is not enough manufacturing capacity out there, and you are in Pennsylvania and we thank you for that. But I wondered if there is anything other than those four points that you would like to make on this?

Mr. HOSBACH. Well, I would really probably like to emphasize the need to get every American to understand the importance of influenza vaccine, being vaccinated. Increasing those inter-pandemic immunization rates will continue to encourage us to expand, as I had mentioned, others to enter the marketplace, and I think you are already seeing some interest from other players. But I think that it is important for several reasons: one, not only for our expansion but that people get used to being immunized; they know who to go to to get immunized, that this becomes a routine and part of their every effort to protect themselves against flu. I think that will help us prepare in the long run for a pandemic.

Mr. ALLEN. Second question, can you talk about how the regulatory process regarding vaccine development and production differs between the U.S. and the E.U.? And part of that question is whether or not more could be done to harmonize the approval processes in the two continents—countries——

Mr. HOSBACH. I am not truly a regulatory expert, and I don't know the specific differences between the E.U. and the U.S., but I do know that there are efforts to harmonize, that much of what they do is similar, and I do know that there is a continuous dialog between the FDA and European Union officials.

Mr. ALLEN. Just one more question for you. Could you elaborate a little bit on the SEC issue? Dr. Gerberding referred to it. I think you mentioned it in your testimony. We are up here trying to figure out what that is all about.

Mr. HOSBACH. Well, you know, it comes from a staff accounting bulletin, which our accounting firms and several accounting firms have interpreted in one way wouldn't allow us to participate or recognize the revenue from the stockpile, so that becomes an issue for us because we would like to have our revenue match our activity.

Mr. ALLEN. So you would only recognize the revenue from the vaccine when the vaccines were used? Is that the——

Mr. HOSBACH. That is correct. And I think this all stems from some of the issues in other larger industries that have had some accounting problems. And so I think that this is a very conservative interpretation, and certainly we need some assistance in clarifying that or perhaps even modifying contracts with CDC that might be able to get around the issue.

Mr. ALLEN. Okay. Thank you. Dr. Crosse, you testified that insufficient hospital and health workforce capacity is an area of concern. Could you give us your characterization of the adequacy of our hospital and health workforce capacity to deal with the next pandemic? And if you can and you think there are gaps—I am sure there are gaps—could you point to specific provisions in the fiscal 2006 budget that are aimed at addressing those gaps?

Ms. CROSSE. I can't give you numbers, but certainly healthcare workforce shortages is a persisting problem. One concern that is especially problematic in a pandemic is that the healthcare workforce would be a highly exposed population and they might themselves become ill or have family members who were ill that they would need to care for. So you might exacerbate any shortages. In this past winter's vaccine shortages, healthcare workforce was not among the priority groups for vaccination, so that would need to be an issue that was considered if you had widespread outbreaks.

There are constant shortages in areas of the country of the nursing workforce. When we did earlier work on bioterrorism preparedness, we found that many communities were planning on surge capacity by calling on their temporary nurse network, but multiple hospitals were counting on the same nurses. And so I think that the bioterrorism funding that has gone to increase hospital planning and preparedness for bioterrorism is helping them to work through some of that planning and to sort through some of the issues. It still doesn't get the bodies there. And the mobile hospitals that were mentioned that could be brought in to be deployed, if you are having nationwide outbreaks, they are still going to have to be staffed locally in all likelihood so that some of the emergency medical care that might be available to be flown in if there was an outbreak in one area would not be available if you had a nationwide pandemic. And so this is a continuing problem.

I can't point to the specific provisions. That would be probably better addressed to the department, but there has been funding through HRSA for hospital preparedness under the bioterrorism funding programs.

Mr. ALLEN. Thank you. The only comment I would add is—this is just an anecdote. I don't mean it as a matter of policy. My son-in-law wants to go to nursing school; he has taken all the prerequisites. He can't get into nursing school until the fall of 2006 in Maine, and it has something to do with the number of slots available. Anyway, thank you all for your testimony. And, Mr. Chairman, I yield back.

Mr. FERGUSON. Mr. Allen, we would be delighted to have your son-in-law in New Jersey if he would like to come to nursing school. Mr. Brown.

Mr. BROWN. I already asked him if he would want to come to New Jersey, and he said he wanted to come to Ohio instead.

Dr. Crosse, I want to follow Mr. Allen's question for a moment and then a question for you, Dr. Iacuzio. Does the bioterrorism funding in some sense, the increase in funding, mask or—maybe mask is a good work—funding for other preparedness for a pandemic outbreak or general public health needs and infrastructure?

Ms. CROSSE. I am not sure what you mean by mask. Is it filling a broader set of needs or do you mean that it——

Mr. BROWN. Or is it looking like it is filling a broader set of needs but in some sense taking away from other public health needs that we have seen?

Ms. CROSSE. I don't think that we have done work recently enough to be able to say how that has played out in the local communities. There are some concerns, I think, that this money coming in may be supplanting some of the funding that otherwise might be provided. But I think it has been providing a broader set of public health preparedness functions than would exist without that funding. It has funded communication systems that are not just used for bioterrorism but for all disease reporting. It has provided some kinds of systems and infrastructure that otherwise might not be in place. I can't speak really to what it has done in terms of whether it has supplanted other funding.

Mr. BROWN. My concern is while CDC funding particularly has not seen major increases in the last few years, unlike NIH which deserved it also, and when there were increases I am not sure that while we did do the right thing certainly for bioterrorism preparedness and answering those issues and preparing local communities, public health officials that we didn't take away from the sort of the workaday infrastructure building and whether it is an issue to like health disparities or whether it is lead poisoning or whether it is nutrition education or whether it is a whole host of issues. But that is more a comment than a question.

Dr. Iacuzio, if I could, according to CDC flu viruses can become resistant to antiviral treatments like Tamiflu. I have done a lot of work on particularly international tuberculosis issues and seen what MDR-TB has done in New York City was our first really horrible experience I think a dozen plus years ago. But we have seen what has happened if we don't follow the DOTS treatment, if patients don't follow the DOTS treatments pretty regularly and pretty precisely, and we know how expensive it is and we know the cure rate, particularly in the most common places for TB, but how the cure rate is pretty difficult and not satisfying when drug resistance occurs. But sticking more to Tamiflu, could you elaborate on the potential and describe how, especially in a pandemic situation, public health officials can best avoid the onset of drug resistance?

Mr. IACUZIO. I believe that the information that we have to date indicates that Tamiflu is safe and effective and there is a low level of resistance. And that has been in published studies. I guess the only thing that I would add is that the data that we do see from places like Japan where they are dosing at a lower dose than has been recommended through the rest of the world and for a shorter duration of time, that probably is the scenario for generating resistance. And there have been a couple of papers that have been published in Japan about increased resistance to antiviral drugs. And it is the same with antibiotics; if you are going to treat, you need to treat with enough antibiotic drug and you need to treat long enough. And if you do the opposite, then you are creating a scenario to generate resistance. I guess that is what I am trying to say. So you need enough drugs in consistent dosing.

Mr. BROWN. Well, I guess this is fairly evident, but you need enough drugs, you need a distribution mechanism to reach remote areas, but to reach them with a large enough supply and with an even-handed distribution and a consistent patient/nurse or patient—whatever the healthcare provider is—relationship that will mean full compliance.

Mr. IACUZIO. Right. And that is why I believe that, you know, discussions of just stockpiling need to go beyond just a big stockpile but actually the whole distribution of how that drug gets out to the individuals who need it.

Mr. BROWN. This is a bit off, but are people with less education typically less likely to be compliant people in a developing world who are not just more remote in terms of distance but less familiar with the healthcare system, all of that? Those would be people likely less compliant——

Mr. IACUZIO. That is——

Mr. BROWN. [continuing] or do we know that?

Mr. IACUZIO. That is a good question that I really—I am not prepared to answer that——

Mr. BROWN. Okay.

Mr. IACUZIO. [continuing] personally.

Mr. BROWN. Okay. Fair enough. All right. Thanks.

Mr. FERGUSON. We are going to do another round of questions if that is all right. I don't think it should take too long. The Chair recognizes himself.

Dr. Hosbach, can you go through the steps and the timeline that it takes for a company from the decision to start, say, an Avian Flu vaccine and actually finishing production in as much detail as you would like? Can you just walk us through from the decision to do that to when it actually is produced and how much time that takes as well?

Mr. HOSBACH. Well, overall, as you heard I think earlier, the process itself will take about 6 months from start to getting doses produced and started to get out the door. The initial steps really are a collaboration with governments and other agencies in terms of identifying that strain, as you indicated, but then getting the reassortant strain that will grow in eggs and start practicing that in our laboratories and also handling it within our manufacturing facility to a point at which it becomes adapted to eggs. From that point on we start producing the vaccine within the egg itself and then activate the virus and harvest the virus from the eggs. I think you will find it interesting that actually the manufacturing piece of it is the smallest portion of the entire chain of production and release. There are large number of release tests, quality standards that need to be met. And actually the release testing those points of quality to observe really take the longest part of the production process. So it is not the actual making it in the eggs that takes long; it is the steps that you have to go through to ensure that you are making a safe and quality and effective product.

Mr. FERGUSON. Where do liability concerns fit into that process? I mean you mentioned a coordinated effort with government at the very beginning. How do liability concerns fit into that process and how do they affect the timeline of being able to produce the product?

Mr. HOSBACH. I think, you know, liability concerns enter in, especially when we are about to enter into something like clinical trials. That is critically important because you are now starting to introduce this into society and introduce this into human subjects. So that becomes one facet of liability that is of concern. But, of course, then once you are ready to release product into the general population, then it is a huge concern because you are not just immunizing perhaps 85 million people; you are immunizing 300 million people.

And I think that if you go back to the mid-'70's, Congress then thought it was important enough in that environment to provide indemnification to companies and to physicians, et cetera. And I think within the current environment that would especially be appropriate. It would put companies in great peril given the unknowns about the actual properties of a new pandemic strain that is a total shift from things that we have utilized before. And given the fact that we only have so few manufacturers, I think you would be putting major assets in harm's way; and not just assets of these pharmaceutical companies, but assets to public health.

Mr. FERGUSON. I am told that, as you referenced in the 1970's with the Swine Flu, that indemnification was a major component to being able to produce a product that was necessary. And as you are leading to, would indemnification hasten that process at all? Would it shorten the timeline to be able to get these products to market?

Mr. HOSBACH. Yes, I think——

Mr. FERGUSON. And we are looking at a——

Mr. HOSBACH. [continuing] in the end-stages it would——

Mr. FERGUSON. And we are looking at a serious problem.

Mr. HOSBACH. In terms of filling and packaging and having the material ready to release, I think that end part of the process could be expedited.

Mr. FERGUSON. Okay. Mr. Brown, did you have any other questions?

Mr. BROWN. A fairly general question, but one that I have not really been satisfied with the answers in the past just because I don't understand it particularly well. We all read about problems with antibiotic resistance. We read about, you know, the way that animals that ranchers and farmers and perhaps veterinarians treat animals prophylactically, partly for growth hormones with antibiotics, partly to protect them prophylactically as the chickens or the cattle are put in small areas. We read about problems obviously with other kinds of antibiotic resistance, physicians over-prescribing, patients demanding when they have a virus they want an antibiotic. I wanted to ask the private sector people here but really any of you to comment. What can Government do to encourage better research and production, getting in the pipeline of antibiotics and antivirals and anti-retrovirals and anti-parasitics?

Mr. PAVIA. Well, I will take that on since, as you know, IDSA has been very involved with that. I think that there are several components to it. One is the limitation of inappropriate use in animal husbandry. And that has come up over and over again. FDA has come up with a process for reviewing that. There is a possibility that antivirals could be used to protect chicken flocks with potential disastrous effects on antiviral resistance if the supplies existed.

The other is education. And there have been efforts to educate patients that have been moderately successful. Educating physicians is another aspect of that. But I think the biggest problem is that we need more agents. Whatever we do to prevent the emergence of resistance or to slow it, it is inevitable. It is the nature of the organisms that they mutate faster than we can develop new drugs. And so we need new agents and we need to continue to do the things that are necessary to have a full pipeline. And to do that we have to understand the profit motives and what it takes to keep a full pipeline.

Mr. TRIPP. I would agree with that. One of our goals is obviously to develop these new breakthrough technologies with Alnylam Pharmaceuticals on RNA interference. These drugs target the actual structural components of the viruses that are very conservative amongst all strains. We have shown these drugs are very effective at targeting and preventing infection of all strains of RSV, for example. And now we are looking at the H5 and H7 strains of influenza. You know, having another tool in your tool belt is the key to preventing resistance. And, of course, following protocol is also important. But I would really recommend that there is more of a linkage in bring private sector companies to the table with current research efforts at universities such as I spoke about today.

Ms. CROSSE. I would just add that we examined this issue of antibiotic resistance from the use of antibiotics in animal feed last year and issued a report with recommendations to FDA to step up its process of review and action on some of the antibiotics of concern. They have taken many years, and we have urged that they speed their process to try to slow down some of these problems from occurring where there is good evidence that resistance is arising from the use among animal flocks. There are other countries who have controls in place and have seen decreases in the prevalence of antibiotic resistance strains among their human population.

Mr. FERGUSON. Just as we close I just want to thank all of our panelists for being here today. There certainly seems to be a consensus that there are serious problems down the road, and we take your exaltations and your advice very seriously and we hope to be taking actions as well. Thank you very much.

[Whereupon, at 1:13 p.m., the subcommittee was adjourned.]

○

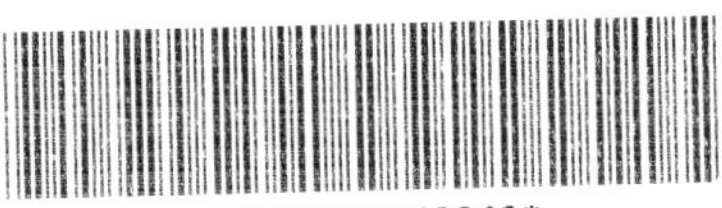

APEX
TP_CF
9780160740046